M000250942

Medical Consultation Pearls

Medical Consultation Pearls

DONNA L. MERCADO, MD, FACP
Assistant Professor
Department of Medicine
Tufts University School of Medicine
Boston, Massachusetts
Director
Medical Consultation Program
Baystate Medical Center
Springfield, Massachusetts

GERALD W. SMETANA, MD, FACP
Assistant Professor
Department of Medicine
Harvard Medical School
Boston, Massachusetts
Herrman L. Blumgart Associate Firm Chief
Division of General Medicine and Primary Care
Beth Israel Deaconess Medical Center
Boston, Massachusetts

HANLEY & BELFUS, INC. / Philadelphia

Publisher: HANLEY & BELFUS, INC.
                Medical Publishers
                210 S. 13th Street
                Philadelphia, PA 19107
                (215) 546-7293, 800-962-1892
                FAX (215) 790-9330
                Website: http://www.hanleyandbelfus.com

Library of Congress Control Number: 2002105214

MEDICAL CONSULTATION PEARLS   ISBN 1-56053-504-0

© 2002 by Hanley & Belfus, Inc. All rights reserved. No part of this book may be reproduced, reused, republished, transmitted in any form or by any means, or stored in a database or retrieval system without written permission of the publisher.

Last digit is the print number: 9 8 7 6 5 4 3 2 1

CONTENTS

Patient

                                                                             Page

1. A 46-year-old woman with respiratory distress after hysterectomy 1
2. A 28-year-old postpartum woman with nausea, vomiting, fever, and tachycardia 4
3. A 62-year-old man with perioperative bleeding 7
4. A 66-year-old man with intraoperative hypotension 9
5. A 41-year-old man with postoperative cardiac arrest 11
6. A 36-year-old man status post liver laceration repair 13
7. A 70-year-old man with chronic obstructive pulmonary disease scheduled for gastrectomy 16
8. A 65-year-old man with schizophrenia, hip fracture, and new postoperative ECG findings 19
9. A 75-year-old woman with chronic obstructive pulmonary disease and fever 4 days after esophagectomy 21
10. A 34-year-old man with asthma scheduled for ventral hernia repair 24
11. A 53-year-old woman scheduled for laparoscopic cholecystectomy 28
12. A 64-year-old man with coronary artery disease scheduled for elective hemicolectomy 32
13. A 53-year-old man with hypertension preparing for elective cervical laminectomy 35
14. An 80-year-old man with aortic stenosis scheduled for transurethral resection of the prostate 39
15. A 63-year-old woman with mitral regurgitation scheduled for elective abdominal hysterectomy 42
16. An 83-year-old man presenting for preoperative medical evaluation before elective cataract surgery 45
17. A 62-year-old woman with depression who is preparing for electroconvulsive therapy 48
18. A 42-year-old woman presenting for preoperative testing before arthroscopic repair of a meniscal tear 51
19. A 77-year-old man presenting for preoperative evaluation before abdominal aortic aneurysm repair 54
20. A 64-year-old woman with a recent myocardial infarction and a new diagnosis of colon cancer 57
21. An 81-year-old woman with chest pain and ECG changes after cholecystectomy 61
22. A 72-year-old man preparing for gastrectomy 64
23. A 67-year-old woman with steroid-requiring polymyalgia rheumatica preparing for total knee replacement 67
24. A 62-year-old man with hypertension in the postanesthesia care unit after elective total hip replacement 70

25. A 64-year-old woman with a productive cough preparing for
    elective hemicolectomy 73

26. A 54-year-old woman with morbid obesity preparing for
    cholecystectomy 76

27. A 73-year-old man with atrial fibrillation after coronary artery
    bypass surgery 79

28. A 42-year-old man with hypertension, headaches, and flushing 83

29. A 48-year-old woman with postoperative agitation and confusion 85

30. A 45-year-old man with recent deep venous thrombosis and new
    lower extremity fractures 88

31. A 72-year-old man with coronary artery disease and chronic
    obstructive pulmonary disease undergoing surgery 90

32. A 50-year-old man with a systolic click undergoing urologic surgery 93

33. A 25-year-old woman at 12 weeks' gestation with hyperglycemia 95

34. A 49-year-old man with severe hypertension after surgery for
    ruptured cerebral aneurysm 98

35. A 33-year-old woman with a history of anorexia nervosa 101

36. A 68-year-old woman with thrombocytopenia undergoing splenectomy 104

37. A 61-year-old man with recent coronary artery stenting, now
    requiring noncardiac surgery 107

38. A 76-year-old woman with Parkinson's disease undergoing
    repair of a fractured hip 109

39. A 67-year-old diabetic man with respiratory arrest after elective surgery 112

40. A 25-year-old pregnant woman with an acute asthmatic exacerbation 115

41. A 38-year-old pregnant woman with unexplained sudden onset of
    dyspnea and chest pain 118

42. A 32-year-old pregnant woman with hypertension presenting at
    33 weeks' gestation 121

43. A 20-year-old pregnant woman with epigastric pain and elevated
    hepatic transaminases 124

44. A 35-year-old man with postoperative excessive urine output 127

45. A 78-year-old man with a history of deep venous thrombosis
    awaiting total knee replacement 130

46. A 77-year-old man with postoperative confusion and agitation 133

47. A 27-year-old pregnant patient with fever, nausea, and abdominal pain 136

48. A 55-year-old man with postoperative agitation and hypertension 139

49. A 73-year-old woman with a myocardial infarction after vascular surgery 142

50. A 69-year-old woman with a permanent cardiac pacemaker requiring
    lumbar laminectomy and fusion for spinal stenosis 145

51. A 72-year-old man with persistent confusion after coronary artery
    bypass graft surgery 147

52. A 58-year-old man with type 2 diabetes mellitus requiring urgent herniorrhaphy 150

53. A 36-year-old man with type 1 diabetes mellitus and an acute abdomen 153

54. A 61-year-old woman on multiple medications presenting for preoperative evaluation 156

55. An 86-year-old woman requiring repair of a hip fracture 159

56. A 47-year-old woman with hypothyroidism, dyspnea, and a postoperative
oxygen requirement 162

57. A 77-year-old man with a postoperative stroke 164

58. A 31-year-old man with intraoperative hemodynamic instability and fever 167

59. A 64-year-old woman with postoperative shortness of breath 170

60. A 40-year-old man with fever and confusion 173

61. An 81-year-old woman with ascending cholangitis and choledocholithiasis 176

62. A 27-year-old woman with a seizure disorder requiring general anesthesia 179

63. A 75-year-old man with confusion and lethargy after a transurethral
resection of the prostate 181

64. A 48-year-old woman with questions about general versus regional anesthesia 184

65. A 45-year-old man with a prosthetic valve who requires a partial lobectomy 187

66. A 78-year-old man with diarrhea after lumbar decompression 190

67. A 26-year-old woman with cirrhosis develops postoperative increase
in abdominal girth 193

68. A 60-year-old woman with abdominal distention and nausea after surgery 196

69. A 62-year-old man with hereditary angioneurotic edema anticipating
mastoidectomy 198

70. A 19-year-old woman with cyanotic heart disease anticipating wisdom
teeth extraction 201

71. A 68-year-old woman with fatigue anticipating cholecystectomy 204

72. A 32-year-old woman with a renal transplant anticipating hysterectomy 207

73. A 66-year-old man with arm deep vein thrombosis 6 days after major
head and neck cancer surgery 210

74. A 79-year-old woman with rheumatoid arthritis and postoperative
respiratory failure 214

75. A 29-year-old man with sickle cell anemia anticipating inguinal herniorrhaphy 217

INDEX 221

CONTENTS BY MEDICAL AREA

Allergy/Immunology   **Page**

   Patient 4 9

   Patient 69 198

Cardiovascular

   Patient 5 11

   Patient 8 19

   Patient 12 32

   Patient 13 35

   Patient 14 39

   Patient 15 42

   Patient 19 54

   Patient 20 57

   Patient 21 61

   Patient 22 64

   Patient 24 70

   Patient 27 79

   Patient 31 90

   Patient 37 107

   Patient 49 142

   Patient 50 145

   Patient 59 170

Endocrinology

   Patient 2 4

   Patient 23 67

   Patient 28 83

   Patient 29 85

   Patient 39 112

   Patient 44 127

   Patient 52 150

   Patient 53 153

   Patient 56 162

   Patient 71 204

Gastroenterology

   Patient 66 190

   Patient 67 193

   Patient 68 196

Geriatrics

Patient 55 159

Patient 61 176

Hematology

Patient 30 88

Patient 36 104

Patient 45 130

Patient 65 187

Patient 73 210

Patient 75 217

Infectious Disease

Patient 25 73

Patient 32 93

Patient 66 190

Patient 70 201

Nephrology

Case 72 207

Neurology

Patient 34 98

Patient 38 109

Patient 46 133

Patient 51 147

Patient 57 164

Patient 62 179

Obstetrics

Patient 33 95

Patient 40 115

Patient 41 118

Patient 42 121

Patient 43 124

Patient 47 136

Psychiatry

Patient 17 48

Patient 35 101

Patient 48 139

Patient 60 173

Pulmonology

Patient 1 1

Patient 6 13

Patient 7 16

Patient 9 21

Patient 10 24

Patient 31 90

Miscellaneous

Patient 3 7

Patient 11 28

Patient 16 45

Patient 18 51

Patient 26 76

Patient 54 156

Patient 58 167

Patient 63 181

Patient 64 184

Patient 74 214

CONTRIBUTORS

Steven L. Cohn, MD, FACP
Chief, Division of General Internal Medicine, Clinical Associate Professor of Medicine, Department of Medicine, SUNY Downstate Medical Center, Brooklyn; Director, Medical Consultation Service, Kings County Hospital, Brooklyn; Associate Medical Director, University Hospital of Brooklyn, New York *Cases 8, 30–32*

Michael Falkenhain, MD
Associate Professor, Department of Clinical medicine, Division of Nephrology, Ohio State University, Columbus, Ohio *Case 73 (coauthor)*

Sean Ian Malone, MD
Clinical Assistant Professor, Department of General Internal Medicine, Wake Forest University, Salisbury, North Carolina *Cases 74, 75 (coauthor)*

Donna L. Mercado, MD, FACP
Assistant Professor, Department of Medicine, Tufts University School of Medicine, Boston; Director, Medical Consultation Program, Baystate Medical Center, Springfield, Massachusetts *Cases 3–5, 33–39, 44–68*

Raymond O. Powrie, MD, FRCP(C), FACP
Associate Professor, Departments of Medicine and Obstetrics/Gynecology, Women and Infants' Hospital, Providence; Educational Director, Division of Obstetric and Consultative Medicine, Brown University School of Medicine, Providence, Rhode Island *Cases 40–43*

Gerald W. Smetana, MD, FACP
Assitant Professor, Department of Medicine, Harvard Medical School, Boston; Herrman L. Blumgart Associate Firm Chief, Division of General Medicine and Primary Care, Beth Israel Deaconess Medical Center, Boston, Massachusetts *Cases 7, 9–27*

Harrison G. Weed, MD, FACP
Associate Professor, Division of General Internal Medicine, Ohio State University College of Medicine, Columbus; Chair, Pharmacy and Therapeutics Committee, The Ohio State University Hospitals, Columbus, Ohio *Cases 69–71, 72 (coauthor), 73, 75 (coauthor)*

Gail A. Welsh, MD, FACP
Assistant Professor, Area of General Internal Medicine, Mayo Medical School, Rochester, Minnesota *Case 2*

Judi Woolger, MD, FACP
Assistant Professor, Division of Internal Medicine, University of Miami School of Medicine, Miami; Director, Medical Consultation Program, Jackson Memorial Hospital, Miami, Florida *Cases 1, 6, 28, 29*

PREFACE

Medical consultation is the art of providing medical advice and problem-solving support for a broad array of medical problems experienced by surgical, obstetric, and psychiatric patients. Over the years, the medical care of these patients has become more complex as the population has aged and presented with increasingly multi-faceted, compound disorders, as maternal age has increased, and as medication management has become more complicated. As a result, medical consultation is becoming more of an art, arguably a medical specialty unto itself, and medical residents in most training programs are now taught details of how medical illness presents and should be managed in this population of patients.

The "pearls" in this book are designed to provide current teaching on the most common and most important medical issues in these patients. The book is especially weighted towards perioperative care, since that is what primary care consultants and hospitalists are most often asked about by their non-medical colleagues.

This book will be useful to medical students, housestaff, medical attendings, and hospitalists; practitioners in anesthesiology and surgery will also find it helpful for practical information on the management of various clinical conditions. The case-based approach makes it uniquely suited to a variety of teaching settings.

Donna L. Mercado, MD, FACP

ACKNOWLEDGMENT

Many thanks to Marie Baez Housey for her invaluable technical and organizational assistance.

DEDICATION

To my children, with all my love:
Austin, Amanda, and Avalon

~ DLM

To Lisa,
For her support, encouragement, and caring

~ GWS

PATIENT 1

A 46-year-old woman with respiratory distress after hysterectomy

A 46-year-old woman, 2 days after uncomplicated hysterectomy and bilateral salpingo-oophorectomy for endometrial cancer, has no complaints. Her respiratory rate is noted to be increased slightly, and her heart rate is 150 beats/min.

Physical Examination: Temperature 99°F, heart rate 125, respirations 26, blood pressure 110/78. Skin: normal. No petechiae. HEENT: normocephalic. Pupils equal. Chest: rapid respirations, lungs clear to auscultation. No wheezing, rales, or rhonchi. Cardiac: tachycardic, normal S_1 and S_2. Grade II/VI systolic murmur over aortic area and left sternal border; no radiation to the neck. Abdomen: soft, distended. Bowel sounds decreased. No rebound or guarding. No organomegaly. Extremities: 1+ edema bilaterally, no Homans's sign. Nontender. Neurologic: awake, oriented. Moves all extremities.

Laboratory Findings: Hct 34%, platelets 160,000/μL. Blood chemistry: normal. ECG: sinus tachycardia, nonspecific ST-T wave changes V4-V6, and presence of $S_1Q_3T_3$ (see Figure). Chest radiograph: no infiltrate, cardiac size normal. ABG: pH 7.44, $PaCO_2$ 40 mmHg, PaO_2 80 mmHg.

Questions: What is the most likely cause for the tachycardia? What other tests should be done?

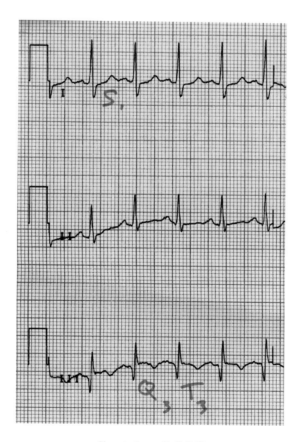

Sinus tachycardia $S_1Q_3T_3$

Diagnosis: Pulmonary embolism (PE) related to postoperative deep venous thrombosis (DVT). Ventilation-perfusion (V/Q) scan or spiral chest CT scan should be done.

Discussion: PE needs to be considered in any patient with unexplained tachycardia or dyspnea. Common predisposing factors include known hypercoagulable state, pregnancy, postoperative state, trauma, and stasis. Cancer, use of oral contraceptives, and long trips also should be considered as causative factors.

Presenting symptoms most commonly are dyspnea or chest pain. Syncope could indicate a central embolus, whereas pleuritic chest pain would indicate a peripheral lesion that irritates the pleural lining. Patients may appear anxious and often have tachycardia. If the embolus is large, blood pressure may drop, or signs of right-sided heart failure may become apparent. The classic triad of $S_1Q_3T_3$ on ECG is actually a relatively rare sign of right heart failure. A more common change would be the development of right bundle-branch block or new T wave inversions on the precordial leads (which indicates right heart strain). Chest radiographs help rule out other conditions that mimic PE, such as pneumothorax or pneumonia, but usually are not diagnostic.

The presence of hypoxemia on ABG is a strong indicator of pulmonary compromise, but studies have shown that at least one in five patients with PE has a normal PaO_2 and normal arterial-alveolar gradient. Abnormal tests with hypoxemia or an increased arterial-alveolar gradient should prompt further investigation. A blood test worth investigation is the D-dimer enzyme-linked immunosorbent assay. If the only D-dimer test available is the latex agglutination test, it is considered inadequate. If the D-dimer is normal (<500 ng/mL), the diagnosis of PE can be ruled out (a normal value excludes PE in 90% of cases). A positive D-dimer is a nonspecific finding in hospitalized patients, however, and it should not be relied on solely to rule in or out a PE.

Options for further testing in a patient with suspected PE include V/Q scan and spiral CT scan. V/Q scan is most useful in a patient who has a relatively normal baseline chest radiograph (the presence of any infiltrates or congestive heart failure makes the reading much less reliable). A high-probability scan usually has at least two areas of perfusion defects in the presence of normal ventilation. An intermediate-probability scan in a patient with high clinical suspicion warrants continued investigation, either with spiral CT or with pulmonary angiography. Although spiral CT is sensitive for larger, more central clots, it is limited in its ability to visualize small vessel or peripheral emboli. Reports of sensitivity and specificity vary widely (53% to 100% sensitivity and 81% to 100% specificity).

Additional studies may include duplex Doppler scans of the lower extremities, but these tend to have low yield in patients with no lower extremity physical findings. Echocardiography can be used to rule out the possibility of congestive heart failure. MRI is excellent at visualizing small vessels but is not yet cost-effective. Contrast pulmonary angiography remains the gold standard.

Studies show that the rate of DVT in patients undergoing non–cancer-related gynecologic surgery who are not given prophylaxis is approximately 6% to 29%, with a PE rate of 0.1% to 0.7%. The rates of DVT and PE in patients undergoing cancer-related gynecologic surgery who are not given prophylaxis are 20% to 38% and 1% to 2%.

The present patient was found to have a high probability V/Q scan consistent with pulmonary embolism. She was treated with supplemental oxygen and full-dose heparin. She made a full recovery and was discharged on warfarin.

Clinical Pearls

1. The main risk factors for DVT and PE include pregnancy, stasis, hypercoagulable state, trauma, and surgery. Other risk factors include cancer, prior DVT and PE, oral contraceptives, and long car or airplane rides.

2. The main signs and symptoms are dyspnea, tachycardia, chest pain, syncope, and pleuritic chest pain. Patients also may be completely asymptomatic. Other warning signs include increased respiratory rate, tachycardia, anxiety, and hemodynamic compromise.

3. The most commonly used modality for diagnosis is V/Q scan, although spiral CT scan is gaining acceptance as a diagnostic tool.

4. A negative D-dimer test, when using the whole blood agglutination assay, is gaining acceptance as a reasonable, noninvasive method of ruling out DVT. The latex agglutination method has a lower sensitivity and specificity, and its interpretation is more subjective.

REFERENCES

1. Wolfe MW, Skibo LD, Goldhaber SZ: Pulmonary embolic disease: Diagnosis, pathophysiologic aspects, and treatment with thrombolytic therapy. Curr Probl Cardiol 10:585–636, 1993.
2. Ferrari E: The ECG in pulmonary embolism: Predictive value of negative T-waves in precordial leads. Chest 111:537–543, 1997.
3. Goldhaber SZ: Diagnosis of pulmonary embolism. Excerpta Medica 2:38–46, 2000.
4. Rathbun SW, Raskob GE, Whitsett, TL et al: Sensitivity and specificity of helical computed tomography in the diagnosis of pulmonary embolism: A systematic review. Ann Int Med 132:227–232, 2000.
5. Davis JD: Prevention, diagnosis, and treatment of venous thromboembolic complications of gynecologic surgery. Am J Obstet Gynecol 184:759–775, 2001.

PATIENT 2

A 28-year-old postpartum woman with nausea, vomiting, fever, and tachycardia

A 28-year-old woman develops nausea, vomiting, fever, and tachycardia 1 day after an emergent cesarean section for fetal distress.

Physical Examination: Temperature 102.3°F, pulse 120, respirations 24, blood pressure 98/52. Skin: diaphoretic. HEENT: normal. Thyroid: diffusely enlarged, nontender. Chest: normal. Cardiac: regular, tachycardic, with I/VI systolic ejection murmur at the left sternal border. Abdomen: normal bowel sounds, nontender, with a clean and dry surgical wound. Extremities: no swelling, erythema, or tenderness. Neuromuscular: tremulous, mildly agitated and confused, oriented to name only. Reflexes brisk with a few beats of clonus bilaterally at the ankles, toes down-going.

Laboratory Findings: Hg 11.0 g/dL, WBC 12,000/μL, platelets normal. Calcium 11.2 mg/dL, alkaline phosphatase 380 U/L, AST 55 U/L, ALT 45 U/L, remaining blood chemistries normal. Thyroid-stimulating hormone <0.01 μU/ml, free thyroxine (T_4) 2.3 μg/dL, triiodothyronine (T_3) 312 ng/dL. Random cortisol 5 μg/dL. ECG: sinus tachycardia. ABG (room air): pH 7.46, $PaCO_2$ 36 mmHg, PaO_2 96 mmHg. Chest radiograph: normal. Urine 23 WBC/high-power field, Gram stain notable for gram-negative rods. Ventilation-perfusion scan: low probability for pulmonary embolus.

Questions: What is the most likely cause of the patient's fever and tachycardia? How would you manage this patient?

Diagnosis and Treatment: Decompensated hyperthyroidism (thyroid storm) precipitated by parturition, surgery, and possible urosepsis. Therapy includes ICU monitoring with supportive care (hydration, nutrition, oxygen, and antipyretics), antithyroid agents (propylthiouracil or methimazole), iodides, β-blockade, corticosteroids, and treatment of urinary tract infection.

Discussion: Thyroid storm is an uncommon condition that usually develops in a patient with poorly controlled hyperthyroidism, although occasionally it can be the initial presentation of previously undiagnosed disease. The cause of thyroid storm is unknown, but precipitating factors include surgery, trauma, parturition, infection, an acute iodine load, diabetic ketoacidosis, or cessation of thyroid medications. A study in 1996 suggested that patients with lower socioeconomic status may be at increased risk.

Thyroid storm is important to recognize because mortality is significant and therapy is lifesaving. The diagnosis is a clinical one because there is no distinction between laboratory values in hyperthyroidism and thyroid storm. In addition to elevations in T_4 and T_3 and leukocytosis, elevation in calcium and alkaline phosphatase (which reflect the effects of thyroid hormone on bone) and nonspecific transaminase elevations may be seen in hyperthyroidism and thyroid storm. Various criteria for diagnosis have been used, but in 1993 Burch developed a point system based on thermoregulatory, cardiovascular, neuropsychiatric, and gastrointestinal dysfunction that helps distinguish between likely thyroid storm, impending storm, and unlikely thyroid storm (see Table).

Point System for Diagnosis of Thyroid Storm*

Thermoregulatory Dysfunction		Cardiovascular Dysfunction	
Temperature (°F)		Tachycardia	
99.0–99.9	5	90–109	5
100–100.9	10	110–119	10
101–101.9	15	120–139	15
102–102.9	20	130–139	20
103–103.9	25	>140	25
> 104	30	Congestive heart failure	
		Mild	5
Central Nervous System Effects		Pedal edema	
Mild	10	Moderate	10
Agitation		Bibasilar rales	
Moderate	20	Severe	15
Delirium		Pulmonary edema	
Psychosis		Atrial fibrillation	10
Extreme lethargy			
Severe	30	**Gastrointestinal/Hepatic Dysfunction**	
Seizure		Moderate	10
Coma		Diarrhea	
		Nausea/vomiting	
Precipitant History		Abdominal pain	
Negative	0	Severe	20
Positive	10	Unexplained jaundice	

*A score of ≥ 45 is highly suggestive of thyroid storm, 25–44 is suggestive of impending storm, < 25 makes thyroid storm unlikely.

Adapted from Burch HB, Wartofsy L: Life-threatening thyrotoxicosis: Thyroid storm. Endocrinol Metab Clin North Am 22:263, 1993.

Therapy may need to be started based on clinical presentation before laboratory values confirm hyperthyroidism. Treatment targets formation and release of thyroid hormone in the gland and peripheral conversion of T_4 to T_3 (see Table). Either propylthiouracil or methimazole is begun initially to inhibit formation of thyroid hormone. Iodinated medications in the form of iopanoic acid, Lugol solution, or saturated solution of potassium iodide (SSKI) prevent release of hormone from the gland. It is important to wait at least 1 hour after the thionamides before administering the iodines because the iodine may be taken up for new hormone if given too soon. Lithium has been used in patients who cannot take thionamides or iodine. Hemodialysis or charcoal hemoperfusion can be used to enhance clearance of thyroid hormone. Graves's disease is a common cause of hyperthyroidism, and these patients can be at increased risk for adrenal insufficiency. Corticosteroids can treat occult adrenal insufficiency and help block peripheral conversion of T_4 to T_3. β-Blockers treat the hyperadrenergic state and may prevent peripheral conversion of T_4 to T_3. Supportive care in the ICU is essential and includes hydration; nutrition with glucose and vitamins; cooling with acetaminophen and cooling blankets; treatment of heart failure and atrial fibrillation, which may develop in many patients; and treatment of the inciting event, if one is found. Acetaminophen is the antipyretic of choice because aspirin may increase thyroid hormone concentrations by interfering with protein binding of T_4 and T_3.

The present patient received initial medication of propylthiouracil and hydrocortisone, 100 mg IV every 8 hours, for associated adrenal insufficiency. Two hours after the propylthiouracil, she received Lugol solution to prevent release of new hormone from the thyroid. Finally, she received propranolol (Inderal), 40 mg every 6 hours, after her blood pressure improved with hydrocortisone and intravenous fluids. Further testing revealed a diagnosis of toxic multinodular goiter.

Treatment of Thyroid Storm

Treatment directed at the thyroid gland
Inhibition of new hormone synthesis
    Thionamide drugs (PTU, methimazole)
Inhibition of thyroid hormone release
    Iodine: iopanoic acid, Lugol solution, SSKI
    Lithium
Treatment directed at peripheral effects of thyroid hormone
Initiation of T_4 to T_3 conversion
    PTU, corticosteroids, β-blockade
        (propranolol, esmolol), iodinated
        radiocontrast agents (iopanoic acid)
Treatment of hyperadrenergic state
    β-blockade
Removal of excess circulating hormone
    Plasmapheresis, charcoal plasma perfusion
Supportive treatment of systemic decompensation
Treatment of hyperthermia
    Acetaminophen, cooling
Correction of dehydration and nutritional deficit
    Fluids and electrolytes, glucose, vitamins
Treatment of heart failure and atrial fibrillation
Treatment of precipitating event

Adapted from Burch HB, Wartofsky L: Life-threatening thyrotoxicosis: Thyroid storm. Endocrinol Metab Clin North Am 22:263, 1993.

Clinical Pearls

1. Thyroid storm is a clinical diagnosis that cannot be distinguished from thyrotoxicosis by laboratory values, but rather by clinical features of thermoregulatory, cardiovascular, neuropsychiatric, and gastrointestinal dysfunction.

2. Thionamides and iodinated medications are the initial treatments directed against thyroid hormone production, but iodines should be delayed for at least 1 hour after thionamides to prevent uptake for new hormone synthesis. Aspirin should not be used as an antipyretic because it can cause decreased protein binding of T_4 and T_3.

3. Therapy may need to be initiated based on clinical presentation before laboratory confirmation of hyperthyroidism. A point system devised by Burch may help determine a strong of likelihood thyroid storm.

REFERENCES
1. Burch HB, Wartofsky L: Life-threatening thyrotoxicosis: Thyroid storm. Endocrinol Metab Clin North Am 22:263, 1993.
2. Sherman SI, Simonson L, Ladenson PW: Clinical and socioeconomic predispositions to complicated thyrotoxicosis: A predictable and preventable syndrome? Am J Med 101:192, 1996.
3. Ringel MD: Management of hypothyroidism and hyperthyroidism in the intensive care unit. Crit Care Clin 17:59–74, 2001.

PATIENT 3

A 62-year-old man with perioperative bleeding

A healthy 62-year-old man presents for total hip replacement for degenerative joint disease. The patient has tolerated prior surgeries (inguinal herniorrhaphy, tooth extraction, and cholecystectomy) without incident. He reports that he is on no medications. Intraoperatively, he has significant unanticipated bleeding requiring transfusion of 2 units of packed RBCs. Postoperatively, his hematocrit continues to drift down, although he does not require additional transfusions.

Physical Examination (Postoperative Day 1): Temperature 99.2°F, pulse 108, respirations 18, blood pressure 98/62. HEENT: normal. Chest: clear. Cardiac: normal. Abdomen: soft, nontender, mildly decreased bowel sounds. No masses. Skin: normal.

Laboratory Findings: WBC 8900/μL, HCT 32%, platelets 154,000/μL, electrolytes normal, INR 1.4, partial thromboplastin time 23 seconds, fibrinogen normal, D-dimer <500, bleeding time 15 minutes.

Question: Why is this patient having bleeding problems now, when prior surgeries were uneventful?

↑ bleeding due to platelet inhibition

- Garlic
- Ginseng
- Ginko
- E.

Diagnosis: Platelet dysfunction secondary to ingestion of herbal medications.

Discussion: On further questioning, the patient revealed that he and his wife had been taking a variety of herbal supplements for the past few months. Use of herbal medications in the United States and elsewhere has become increasingly common. A recent survey found that during their preoperative assessments, more than 70% of patients failed to reveal their use of herbal medications. It has been noted in other studies that patients do not disclose their use of herbal remedies unless specifically asked. There are several possible explanations. Some patients believe that their physicians are not knowledgeable about the use of herbal medications or disapprove of their use. Some patients do not regard them as medications and do not think that these agents affect their medical care. It is important to ask patients specifically about the use of herbal medications preoperatively.

Herbal medications can affect perioperative care in a variety of ways: via direct pharmacologic action, via alteration of the action of other drugs at the effector sites, and via alteration of the pharmacokinetics (absorption, distribution, metabolism, and elimination) of other drugs. According to a recent survey, the most commonly used herbal medications are echinacea, ginkgo biloba, St. John's wort, garlic, and ginseng. Another survey mentioned three additional herbals: ephedra, kava, and valerian. Of these herbal medications, three have the potential to increase bleeding risk: garlic, ginkgo biloba, and ginseng.

Garlic causes dose-dependent inhibition of platelet aggregation. It also may potentiate the effect of other platelet inhibitors. Because the effects are possibly irreversible, garlic should be stopped at least 7 days preoperatively.

Ginkgo inhibits platelet-activating factor. Although small clinical trials did not reveal bleeding complications, there are sporadic cases in the literature of spontaneous bleeding and postoperative bleeding. The terpenoid components of the ginkgo are responsible for the risk of bleeding. Based on a half-life of 3 to 10 hours, ginkgo should be stopped at least 3 days preoperatively.

Ginseng is believed to inhibit platelet aggregation, likely in an irreversible fashion. It should be stopped at least 7 days preoperatively. Ginseng also is associated with a decrease in the effectiveness of warfarin (Coumadin).

Vitamin E is used commonly by the general population, and it is associated with effects on platelet aggregation and potentiation of the anticoagulation effects of warfarin. Because its effect on platelet aggregation may be irreversible, vitamin E should be stopped at least 7 days before surgery.

Of the other commonly used herbal medications, valerian and kava, can potentiate the sedative effects of anesthetics. Ephedra can cause myocardial ischemia, stroke, and significant interactions with monoamine oxidase inhibitors. It also can cause intraoperative hemodynamic instability in patients who have used it for a long time. St. John's wort caused induction of the cytochrome P-450 system, affecting the metabolism of multiple drugs.

The present patient admitted to use of high-dose vitamin E, ginkgo biloba, garlic, and a multiherbal product, of which he had no idea of the components. He did not stop any of these preoperatively and still was taking them in the hospital. He also had been taking over-the-counter ibuprofen (Advil) but had not reported this. His increased need for transfusion intraoperatively was believed to be due in large part to these multiple agents.

Clinical Pearls

1. All patients should be asked specifically whether or not they use herbal products.

2. Because the full perioperative effects of herbal medications are not yet known, some practitioners stop all these agents 2 weeks preoperatively.

3. To date, herbal medications have been responsible for perioperative myocardial infarction, stroke, bleeding, inadequate oral anticoagulation, prolonged or inadequate anesthesia, and organ transplant rejection.

REFERENCES

1. Bovill JG: Adverse drug interactions in anesthesia. J Clin Anesth 9(suppl 6):35–135, 1997.
2. Kaye AD, Clarke RC, Sabar R, et al: Herbal medications: Current trends in anesthesiology practice—a hospital survey. J Clin Anesth 12:468–471, 2000.
3. Tsen LC, Segal S, Pothier M, Bader AM: Alternative medicine use in presurgical patients. Anesthesiology 93:148–151, 2000.
4. Ang-Lee MK, Moss J, Yuan CS: Herbal medicines and perioperative care. JAMA 286:208–216, 2001.

PATIENT 4

A 66-year-old man with intraoperative hypotension

A 66-year-old man with severe degenerative joint disease presents for left total knee replacement. His past medical history is notable for hypertension, and his preoperative evaluation is unremarkable. Intraoperatively, he becomes unstable, with sudden hypotension (70 mmHg systolic) and an increase in heart rate to 144 beats/min.

Physical Examination (Immediately Postoperatively): Temperature 98.1°F, pulse 102, respirations 22, blood pressure 98/58. Chest: clear. Cardiac: no jugular venous distention. Regular rhythm. Normal S_1 and S_2 without murmur, rub, or gallop. Abdomen: normal. Neurologic: awake and oriented. No focal findings.

Laboratory Findings: WBC 10,200/μL, Hct 33%, electrolytes normal, troponin <0.3. ECG: sinus tachycardia with nonspecific ST-T wave changes in the lateral leads. Chest radiograph: unremarkable.

Questions: What is the cause of the patient's intraoperative hypotension? What diagnostic studies should be performed?

Answers: Intraoperative anaphylaxis. The immediate diagnostic study is serum tryptase level. Postoperative diagnostic studies are intradermal skin testing and radioimmunoassay antibody testing.

Discussion: Intraoperative hypotension can be caused by a variety of clinical entities, such as hemorrhage, insufficient intravenous volume, anesthetic agents, myocardial ischemia, cardiogenic shock, valvular disease (i.e., aortic stenosis), sepsis, pulmonary embolism, venous air embolism, hypothyroidism, adrenal insufficiency, and anaphylaxis. Immediate intraoperative assessment of the patient's physical examination, ECG, and hematocrit sometimes reveals a cause. Reassessment of the patient's history looking for clues that would point to hypothyroidism, adrenal insufficiency, infection, or allergy also can be helpful. The clinician should maintain a high index of suspicion of intraoperative anaphylaxis if the cause for the intraoperative instability is not immediately evident.

Intraoperative anaphylaxis is thought to occur with an incidence of 1 case per 5000 to 25,000 anesthetics, although the rate may be higher because some episodes undoubtedly are not recognized. The mortality rate is reported as 3.4%. It usually is caused by intravenous medications, although other culprits are latex, blood transfusions, preoperative medications, and implantable prosthetic devices. Cardiovascular signs of anaphylaxis include hypotension, tachycardia, dysrhythmias, pulmonary hypertension, and cardiac arrest. Other signs include urticaria, laryngeal edema, wheezing, flushing, and angioedema. At times, the only clue in the anesthetized patient is hypotension.

Diagnosis of anaphylaxis usually is made on clinical grounds, sometimes supported by skin test results or radioimmunoassay antibody test results, obtained after the incident. Serum tryptase level, if drawn within 20 minutes of the acute event, usually is elevated and can be helpful in confirming the diagnosis.

The present patient became hypotensive shortly after he was exposed intraoperatively to the knee prosthesis that was being placed. The prosthesis had been washed in bacitracin solution before placement, and the surgical area had been irrigated with the same solution. The patient had been exposed to bacitracin previously during a prior joint surgery.

The patient was stabilized with fluids and ephedrine, followed by epinephrine and dopamine. After 30 minutes, temporary joint stabilizers were placed. The patient was transferred to the ICU, but the rest of his postoperative course was uneventful. After initial stabilization, the patient did well and had no further reactions during hospitalization. Because it was unclear what the patient had reacted to and because he needed completion of joint replacement, he underwent allergic testing as an outpatient to the various medications he had been exposed to. The only one he reacted to was bacitracin. The patient subsequently underwent successful completion of the total knee replacement without bacitracin.

Clinical Pearls

1. Intraoperative anaphylaxis usually presents with a variety of cardiovascular and peripheral findings, but at times it presents only as resistant hypotension. A high index of suspicion must be maintained.

2. Latex allergy is growing in incidence. Individuals at higher risk include health care workers; patients with a history of multiple surgeries; patients with spina bifida; and patients with food allergies to banana, avocado, and kiwi.

3. Other common medications causing intraoperative allergy include narcotics, muscle relaxants, protamine, antibiotics, barbiturates, and local anesthetics—generally the *esters* (chloroprocaine, procaine, tetracaine, cocaine, benzocaine) and not the *amides* (bupivacaine, lidocaine, dibucaine, mepivacaine).

REFERENCES
1. Currie M, Webb RK, Williamson JA, et al: Clinical anaphylaxis: An analysis of 2000 incident reports. Anaesth Intensive Care 21:621–625, 1993.
2. Blas M, Briesacher KS, Lobato EB: Bacitracin irrigation: A cause of anaphylaxis in the operating room. Anesth Analg 91:1027–1028, 2000.
3. Foxell RM: Incidence of anaphylaxis under anesthesia. Anesthesia 56:294–295, 2001.

PATIENT 5

A 41-year-old man with postoperative cardiac arrest

A 41-year-old, healthy man undergoes anteroposterior fusion for L4–5. The patient has a 24-pack-year tobacco history but quit smoking 1 year before surgery. He ran 10 miles per day before a back injury 2 years before the time of surgery without cardiopulmonary symptoms. After the back injury, he could walk 1.5 miles per day without symptoms. One day postoperatively, the patient is noted to be doing well; his only complaint is pain at the surgical site. Twenty minutes after morning rounds are done, he is found by the nurse to be pulseless and without respirations. He undergoes advanced cardiac life support and is found to be in asystole.

Physical Examination: Temperature 99.6°F, heart rate 127, respirations 14 by Ambu-bag, blood pressure 90/52. Skin: no urticaria, no lesions. Chest: clear to auscultation. Cardiac: regular tachycardia without gallops or murmurs. Abdomen: normal. Extremities: no edema. Neurologic: unresponsive to pain. No spontaneous movement of extremities. No gag reflex. Pupils minimally reactive. Intact doll's eyes reflexes. Deep tendon hyperreflexia.

Laboratory Findings: CBC: WBC 11,400/μL without a left shift, Hct 34%, platelets 215,000/μL, chemistries normal. ABG (during advanced cardiac life support): pH 7.19, PO_2 112 mmHg, PCO_2 47 mmHg, lactate 8.9 mg/dL, troponin <0.3 μg/L. Tryptase level normal. ECG: sinus tachycardia without changes from preoperative ECG.

Question: What is the most likely cause of the patient's cardiac arrest?

Diagnosis: Postoperative cardiac arrest. The differential diagnosis for postoperative cardiac arrest includes dysrhythmia, myocardial infarction, pulmonary embolism, autonomic dysfunction, and anaphylaxis.

Discussion: Benign ventricular dysrhythmias are common perioperatively, but it is rare for them to lead to sustained ventricular tachycardia, ventricular fibrillation, and death. Postoperatively, even after cardiac procedures, atrial dysrhythmias are the most common. Ventricular dysrhythmias are rare and can be due to a prolonged Q-T interval (secondary to hypokalemia, hypomagnesemia, β-agonist therapy, diabetes, or hereditary conditions), cardiac ischemia, or ventricular irritability. Postoperative catecholamines can incite ventricular irritability in patients with abnormal myocardium in conditions such as cardiomyopathies and occult coronary artery disease. Sometimes no specific cause can be found.

Autonomic insufficiency can cause sudden postoperative respiratory or cardiac arrest in patients with primary dysautonomias and in patients with diabetic neuropathy who have autonomic involvement. The arrest generally occurs intraoperatively or within a few hours of surgery; there is no prophylactic treatment available except watchful waiting.

Postoperative anaphylaxis can occur to any medication or substance but especially latex, antibiotics, nonsteroidal agents, and narcotics. A tryptase level drawn within 20 minutes of the event should be elevated. If anaphylaxis is suspected, patients should have the offending agents discontinued and should receive histamine 1 and 2 receptor blockers (i.e., loratadine and ranitidine) and steroids.

In an unresponsive patient, pulmonary embolism can be diagnosed by spiral CT scan or by angiogram. D-Dimer testing is nonspecific in the setting of acute illness and is not useful in this circumstance.

The present patient responded to epinephrine and lidocaine; sinus rhythm was restored. He was ventilated easily and had a prompt pulmonary response to oxygen; he had a negative pulmonary angiogram, a normal tryptase level, a normal echocardiogram, negative cardiac enzymes, a normal head CT scan, normal chemistries, and a normal ECG. He was not diabetic and had no evidence of autonomic insufficiency. He was believed to have had idiopathic ventricular irritability versus occult coronary artery disease with secondary ventricular irritability. An electroencephalogram was consistent with severe hypoxic cerebral damage, and his family removed him from life support.

Clinical Pearls

1. Postoperative ventricular tachycardia occurs most often in the setting of preexisting coronary artery disease, cardiomyopathy, or metabolic derangements and rarely occurs in the absence of these.

2. Preoperative frequent premature ventricular contractions on ECG is generally a benign condition; occult ischemic disease should be investigated in older patients or patients with significant cardiac risk factors. Suppressive antiarrhythmics are not necessary.

3. Autonomic neuropathy can be present in patients with long-standing diabetes and has a low risk of causing sudden cardiac or respiratory arrest in the immediate postoperative period.

REFERENCES

1. Page MMcB, Watkins PJ: Cardiorespiratory arrest and diabetic autonomic neuropathy. Lancet 1:14–16, 1978.
2. Davies MJ, Thomas AC: Plaque fissuring—the cause of acute myocardial infarction, sudden ischemic death, and crescendo angina. Br Heart J 53:363, 1985.
3. O'Kelly B, Browner WS, Massie B, et al: Ventricular arrhythmias in patients undergoing noncardiac surgery. JAMA 268:217–221, 1992.
4. Weitz HM: Arrhythmias and conduction disturbances. In Lubin MF, Walker HK, Smith RB (eds): Medical Management of the Surgical Patient, 3rd ed. Philadelphia, J.B. Lippincott, 1995.

PATIENT 6

A 36-year-old man status post liver laceration repair

A 36-year-old man suffers a liver laceration injury during a motor vehicle accident. He undergoes repair of the laceration. On postoperative day 2, he is found on rounds to be tachycardic, hypoxic, and confused.

Physical Examination: Temperature 102.4°F, heart rate 140, respirations 34, blood pressure 116/60. Skin: scattered ecchymosis from trauma. Scattered axillary petechiae. HEENT: Normocephalic. Pupils equal and reactive to light. Fundi: occasional Hollenhorst plaques. Cardiac: tachycardic S_1, S_2. No murmurs or rubs. Chest: shallow, rapid breathing, bilateral coarse rhonchi. Abdomen: soft, nontender, no rebound or guarding. Extremities: no edema. Neurologic: confused; disoriented to person, place, and time. Responsive to pain, moves all extremities, agitated.

Laboratory Findings: Hct 30%, platelets 74,000/μL, blood chemistries normal. ECG: sinus tachycardia, no ischemic changes. Chest radiograph: new patchy pulmonary infiltrates. (Admission radiograph with no infiltrates, no pneumothorax.) ABG: pH 7.50, $PaCO_2$ 30 mmHg, PaO_2 48 mmHg (no prior ABG to compare). Ventilation-perfusion scan: negative for pulmonary embolism. Pelvic and femoral films: bilateral pelvic rami fractures.

Questions: What is the most likely cause for the rapid deterioration of the patient? What other physical examination findings might be present? What additional tests should be performed? What is the most appropriate therapy?

Answers: The most likely cause is fat embolism syndrome. Physical exam findings may include tachypnea; tachycardia; fever; rales or rhonchi; retinal emboli (Hollenhorst plaques); fleeting petechiae across chest, axillae, neck, and conjunctivae; central nervous system depression after initial restlessness; urinary incontinence; focal seizures. Additional tests are urinalysis with fat globules, cryostat of frozen section of blood to stain for fat, transcranial Doppler to detect microemboli. Treatment is primarily supportive.

Discussion: Fat emboli and fat embolism syndrome are a major cause of morbidity and mortality, especially in patients with fractures or multiple injuries. Fat embolism syndrome also has been found in association with multiple other nontraumatic disease processes, such as collagen vascular diseases, diabetes, burns, neoplasms, blood transfusions, cardiopulmonary bypass, and severe infection. Prompt recognition is important because of the known association with acute respiratory distress.

Recognition of fat embolism syndrome is difficult primarily because it is often a diagnosis of exclusion. As described in the present patient, typical features include complaints of shortness of breath, restlessness, and confusion followed by rapid neurologic deterioration. Patients may develop fever to 102°F, tachypnea to rates of 30 breaths/min or more, and rapidly resolving petechiae. Retinal fat emboli located at bifurcations of vessels are seen occasionally on funduscopic examination. These appear as bright, refractile bodies and are termed *Hollenhorst plaques*. They often are fleeting in nature. There is a wide spectrum of presentations, however, and patients simply may have tachypnea, hypoxemia, and tachycardia, often resembling the presentation of pulmonary embolus.

Although there is no pathognomonic test for fat embolism syndrome, arterial hypoxemia is central to making the diagnosis and can be followed to monitor response to therapy. A useful set of diagnostic criteria is that established by Gurd in 1970. Based on that definition, major clinical criteria for the diagnosis of fat embolism syndrome include hypoxia (PO_2 <60 mmHg and FiO_2 >0.4), central nervous system depression, and petechiae. Minor clinical criteria include tachycardia (heart rate >120 beats/min), fever (temperature >102°F), thrombocytopenia (platelet count <150,000/μL), fat globules in the urine or sputum, retinal emboli, and anemia that cannot be accounted for by another clinical explanation. To meet the criteria for clinical diagnosis, patients must have at least one major sign and three minor signs or two major and two minor signs. Therapy consists primarily of supportive care. Maintaining airway, restoring blood volume (and blood products if anemia or thrombocytopenia is severe), and restoring electrolyte balance are imperative. Immobilizing any injured limbs before transfers is important to avoid excessive movement, which might lead to further fat embolization.

Treatment of hypoxemia depends on the severity of the case. Oxygen can be administered by facemask, nasal cannula, or endotracheal intubation. Other considerations for therapy include ethanol, heparin, hypertonic glucose, and corticosteroids, but none of these has been proven consistently to improve outcomes.

Mortality from fat emboli or fat embolism syndrome is estimated at 7%, with outcome depending on severity of the syndrome and associated injuries or conditions (see Table). Diagnosis is difficult because of the overlap of signs and symptoms found in most trauma patients. The clinician needs to maintain a high level of suspicion and rapidly institute supportive measures aimed at respiratory support.

Conditions Associated With Fat Embolism

Trauma Related	Non–Trauma Related
Long bone fractures	Pancreatitis
Pelvic fractures	Diabetes mellitus
Orthopedic procedures	Infection
Burns	Sickle cell disease
	Alcoholic liver disease
	Neoplasms
	Anesthesia

The present patient required intubation and ventilatory support for 8 days. His infiltrates initially worsened, then cleared slowly over 18 days. His neurologic condition improved over 1 week; respiratory and neurologic abnormalities resolved by the time of discharge.

Clinical Pearls

1. Fat embolism syndrome usually manifests 24 to 72 hours after the initial insult (the proposed mechanism of disease suggests degradation of the embolized fat into free fatty acids, which then causes an adult respiratory distress syndrome–like syndrome).

2. Classic triad for presentation is hypoxemia, neurologic changes, and petechial rash, usually in that order: Respiratory distress presents first, followed by confusion, and fleeting petechial rash.

3. The petechial rash is considered pathognomonic and occurs in approximately 20% to 50% of cases.

4. Treatment is supportive. Historical use of ethanol, heparin, albumin, or hypertonic glucose solutions has not shown consistent benefit. Use of intravenous corticosteroids shows some potential benefits, although human trials have been small and poorly controlled.

REFERENCES

1. Gurd A: Fat embolism: An aid to diagnosis. J Bone Joint Surg Br 52:732–737, 1970.
2. Levy DL: The fat embolism syndrome: A review. Clin Orthop 261:281–286, 1990.
3. Francis CW: Fat embolism syndrome/acute respiratory distress syndrome. In Fractures in Adults, 4th ed. 1996, pp 433–443.
4. Bulger EM, et al: Fat embolism syndrome: A ten year review. Arch Surg 132:435–439, 1997.

[Handwritten notes:]

"Clinical": hypoxia ①
petechia ③
↓ CNS ②

~24 → 72 p̄ initial trauma

tachy
fever
↓ platelets

fat embolized
→ degraded to FFA
→ ARDS

PATIENT 7

A 70-year-old man with chronic obstructive pulmonary disease scheduled for gastrectomy

A 70-year-old man presents to the preoperative testing area for evaluation before a planned partial gastrectomy for adenocarcinoma in the gastric antrum. He has a 40-year history of cigarette smoking, averaging two packs per day. He has been admitted to the hospital an average of once each year for the treatment of exacerbations of chronic obstructive pulmonary disease (COPD); his last admission was 2 months ago. At baseline, he is dyspneic after one block of walking on level ground or one flight of stairs. He has a daily nonproductive cough. His current symptoms are similar to baseline, and he has had no recent increase in his usual dyspnea or cough. Past medical history includes degenerative arthritis of both hips and type 2 diabetes. Current medications are ipratropium and albuterol metered-dose inhalers, ibuprofen, and glyburide.

Physical Examination: Temperature 98°F, heart rate 90, respirations 16, blood pressure 140/90. General appearance: Thin, chronically ill man in mild respiratory distress at rest and using accessory neck muscles of respiration. Chest: diffuse decrease in breath sounds, inspiratory-to-expiratory ratio of 1:3, mild diffuse expiratory wheezes. Cardiac: regular rhythm, normal S_1 and S_2 with a soft S_4. Jugular venous pressure normal.

Laboratory Findings: Hct 50%, WBC 7200/μL. ECG: normal sinus rhythm at 82, right-axis deviation. Chest radiograph (see Figure): hyperinflation, flattened hemidiaphragms, and increased interstitial markings at the bases.

Question: What is the patient's risk for postoperative pulmonary complications?

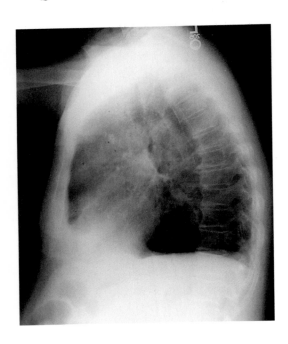
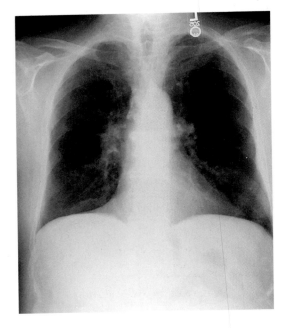

Answer: COPD is a major risk factor for postoperative pulmonary complications.

Discussion: Postoperative pulmonary complications are more frequent than postoperative cardiac complications and contribute equally to morbidity, mortality, and length of hospital stay. Important postoperative pulmonary complications include pneumonia, exacerbation of underlying COPD, prolonged mechanical ventilation, and atelectasis. Patient-related and procedure-related factors contribute to risk. COPD is the strongest predictor of postoperative pulmonary complications among patient-related risk factors. The relative risk associated with COPD ranges from 2.7 to 4.7. The degree of risk varies proportionately with the severity of the underlying lung disease. Among patients with equal severity of COPD, a greater risk exists for current smokers than for patients who have not smoked for at least 2 months. Poor functional class, as defined by exercise capacity or the American Society of Anesthesiologists' classification, is also a risk factor in patients with COPD.

In patients with COPD, the highest risk surgeries are those involving the chest and upper abdomen because of splinting, diaphragmatic dysfunction, and decreased lung volumes after surgery. Additional procedure-related risk factors include surgery lasting longer than 3 hours, the use of general anesthesia, and the use of pancuronium as a neuromuscular blocking agent.

The role of pulmonary function testing to stratify risk for patients with COPD is controversial. One could argue for the use of routine preoperative spirometry if it either stratified risk more effectively than clinical evaluation or identified patients for whom the risk of surgery was prohibitive. Studies suggest, however, that spirometry does not meet either of these goals. In one report, clinical factors, including decreased breath sounds, prolonged expiration, rales, rhonchi, wheezes, high score on the Goldman or Charlson risk indices, and an abnormal chest radiograph, predicted postoperative pulmonary complications to a greater degree than the results of spirometry. In another study, smokers undergoing abdominal surgery who had abnormal spirometry were compared with matched patients with normal spirometry. Although there was an increase in bronchospasm among the patients with abnormal spirometry, there was no difference between the two groups in the incidence of prolonged intubation, pneumonia, prolonged ICU stay, or death.

Patients identified as high risk by spirometry can undergo surgery with an acceptable degree of risk. In a study of 107 surgeries in patients with COPD and a FEV_1 of less than 50% of predicted, there was only one death among noncoronary procedures, and the incidence of moderate or severe pulmonary complications was 24%.

Routine preoperative spirometry does not add significantly to the risk assessment. Clinicians should obtain spirometry for patients with COPD if, after clinical evaluation, it is not clear whether the patient is at his or her best baseline level of function. Spirometry should not be used to deny surgery because there is no prohibitive value below which the risk is unacceptable.

The present patient is at high risk for postoperative pulmonary complications because of his history of poor exercise capacity; the upper abdominal incision; and the physical findings of decreased breath sounds, wheezing, and prolonged expiratory phase. Spirometry would confirm this risk stratification but would be unlikely to change the risk assessment.

Clinical Pearls

1. COPD is the most important patient-related risk factor for postoperative pulmonary complications.

2. Current smokers and recent quitters have a higher risk of pulmonary complications than patients who have stopped smoking for at least 8 weeks.

3. Upper abdominal and thoracic surgeries carry the greatest risk for pulmonary complications in patients with COPD.

4. Routine preoperative spirometry does not predict pulmonary complications more accurately than clinical evaluation alone.

REFERENCES

1. Kroenke K, Lawrence VA, Theroux JF, Tuley MR: Operative risk in patients with severe obstructive pulmonary disease. Arch Intern Med 152:967–971, 1992.
2. Lawrence VA, Hilsenbeck SG, Mulrow CD, et al: Incidence and hospital stay for cardiac and pulmonary complications after abdominal surgery. J Gen Intern Med 10:671–678, 1995.
3. Lawrence VA, Dhanda R, Hilsenbeck SG, Page CP: Risk of pulmonary complications after elective abdominal surgery. Chest 110:744–750, 1996.
4. Warner DO, Warner MA, Offord KP, et al: Airway obstruction and perioperative complications in smokers undergoing abdominal surgery. Anesthesiology 90:372–379, 1999.
5. Smetana GW: Preoperative pulmonary evaluation. N Engl J Med 340:937–944, 1999.

PATIENT 8

A 65-year-old man with schizophrenia, hip fracture, and new postoperative ECG findings

A 65-year-old man is admitted to the hospital after falling sustaining a hip fracture. The patient is schizophrenic and mute, refusing to answer any questions about his fall or his past medical history. His aide states that he tripped but did not lose consciousness. The only medical problem she is aware of is a history of hypertension. He is taking diuretic and antipsychotic medications. The patient is taken to the operating room for an open reduction and internal fixation of the fracture. Intraoperatively, he develops respiratory distress and is given furosemide. A Swan-Ganz catheter is inserted, and the pulmonary capillary wedge pressure is 19 mmHg. The patient remains stable, and he subsequently is taken to the recovery room.

Physical Examination: Temperature 99°F, pulse 110, respirations 22, blood pressure 140/80. HEENT: normal. Neck: no jugular venous disease, normal carotid pulses without bruits. Heart: normal heart sounds, II/6 systolic murmur at the left sternal border, no gallop. Chest: few bibasilar rales. Abdomen: normal. Extremities: no edema or calf tenderness, right lower extremity tender to palpation at the surgical site. Neurologic: no focal deficits. Cannot assess mental status, but patient is awake and alert, refusing to respond to questions.

Laboratory Findings: CBC: normal. Blood chemistries: normal. Chest radiograph: mild pulmonary vascular congestion, no cardiomegaly. Preoperative ECG: normal sinus rhythm with left anterior hemiblock, no Q waves or ischemic changes. Cardiac enzymes: pending. ABG: pH 7.44, PO_2 97, PCO_2 34 (on 2 L of oxygen via nasal cannula). Postoperative ECG (see Figure): sinus tachycardia with left anterior hemiblock, right bundle-branch block, nonspecific ST-T wave changes, and unifocal premature ventricular contractions (PVCs).

Questions: What is the diagnosis of ECG findings? Does the patient need a pacemaker? Is antiarrhythmic therapy indicated?

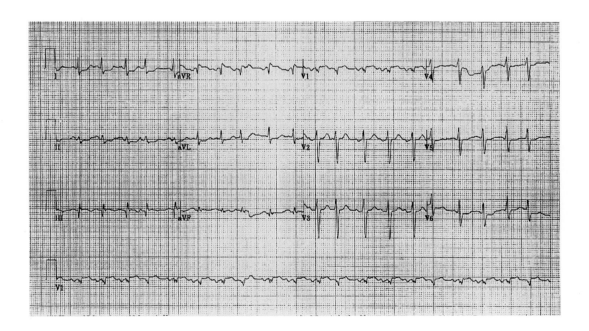

Diagnosis and Treatment: New right bundle-branch block and PVCs in a patient with possible cardiac disease. The isolated PVCs do not require treatment.

Discussion: New conduction defects or arrhythmias in the perioperative period may result from many conditions. In the present case, it is crucial to determine when the right bundle-branch block occurred. If it happened immediately after insertion of the Swan-Ganz catheter, the catheter is the likely culprit. If it occurred before or much later, other causes need to be considered, including **myocardial ischemia** or **infarction** and **pulmonary embolism**. Other diseases associated with development of a new right bundle-branch block include congestive heart failure, pericarditis or myocarditis, exacerbation of chronic obstructive pulmonary disease, or rate-related bundle-branch block. Right bundle-branch block also can be found in hypertensive heart disease, cardiomyopathy, rheumatic or congenital heart disease, and cardiac tumors.

The present patient did not have any past history of cardiac disease, although he had cardiac risk factors, being a 65-year-old man with hypertension. The intraoperative respiratory distress could be secondary to iatrogenic fluid overload, myocardial ischemia or infarction, congestive heart failure, pulmonary embolism, or chronic obstructive pulmonary disease. He responded to treatment with diuretics, then was noted to have these new ECG changes. The first set of cardiac enzymes was reported as normal, and the patient remained asymptomatic with a bifascicular block.

Swan-Ganz catheters can cause a right bundle-branch block in 1% to 5% of cases, and if the patient had preexisting left bundle-branch block, this could result in a trifascicular or complete heart block necessitating placement of a temporary pacemaker. A myocardial infarction eventually was ruled out. Although pulmonary embolism may be difficult to exclude, it is less likely to occur immediately postoperatively in a patient with no prior risk factors who was ambulatory. Respiratory alkalosis with mild hypoxemia is seen commonly in the postoperative period. The isolated PVCs, even associated with myocardial infarction, do not require treatment; however, should the patient develop ventricular tachycardia in this setting, antiarrhythmic therapy would be warranted. In the present patient, the Swan-Ganz catheter was pulled back slowly, and the right bundle-branch block resolved, as did the PVCs.

Clinical Pearls

1. Myocardial ischemia or infarction should be considered in all patients who develop perioperative congestive heart failure, arrhythmias, or conduction abnormalities.

2. Asymptomatic bifascicular blocks do not require prophylactic pacing before surgery.

REFERENCES

1. Thompson IR, Dalton BC, Lappas DG, Lowenstein E: Right bundle branch block and complete heart block caused by the Swan-Ganz catheter. Anesthesiology 51:359–362, 1979.
2. O'Kelly B, Browner WS, Massie B, et al: Ventricular arrhythmias in patients undergoing noncardiac surgery. JAMA 268:217–221, 1992.
3. Gauss A, Hubner C, Radermacher P, et al: Perioperative risk of bradyarrhythmias in patients with asymptomatic chronic bifascicular block or left bundle branch block. Anesthesiology 88:679–687, 1998.

PATIENT 9

A 75-year-old woman with chronic obstructive pulmonary disease and fever 4 days after esophagectomy

A 75-year-old woman presents with fever 4 days after esophagectomy for a squamous cell carcinoma. She has smoked two packs of cigarettes per day for 50 years and continues to smoke. She has been hospitalized for exacerbations of chronic obstructive pulmonary disease (COPD) three times within the past year. At baseline, she is dyspneic with mild exertion, such as walking from one room to the next in her home. She has a chronic daily cough productive of yellow sputum. She notes no recent change in her dyspnea or exercise capacity. She does not require long-term oxygen administration. Her past medical history includes hypertension. Medications on admission include albuterol metered-dose inhaler, ipratropium inhaler, theophylline, and hydrochlorothiazide.

Physical Examination: Temperature 98.0°F orally, heart rate 80, respirations 16, blood pressure 150/86. General appearance: chronically ill appearing in mild respiratory distress at rest using pursed-lip breathing. HEENT: normal. Chest: increased anteroposterior diameter, moderate decrease in breath sounds diffusely. Inspiratory-to-expiratory ratio of 1:3, scattered wheezes, no rales or rhonchi. Cardiac: regular rhythm, normal S_1, accentuated P_2, no murmurs. Jugular venous pulse 6 cm. Extremities: trace edema to the midcalf bilaterally.

Laboratory Findings: Hct 49%, WBC 9400/μL with a normal differential. SMA-7 normal. ECG: sinus rhythm at 84, P pulmonale, right-axis deviation, otherwise normal. Admission chest radiograph: hyperinflation and flattened diaphragms consistent with emphysema.

Hospital Course: Patient underwent a distal esophagectomy. She required prolonged mechanical ventilation for the first 2 days after surgery. On the fourth postoperative day, her temperature rose to 102.4°F orally, and she developed an increase in sputum production. Her chest radiograph is shown (see Figure).

Question: How might you have reduced the risk of postoperative pulmonary complications in this patient?

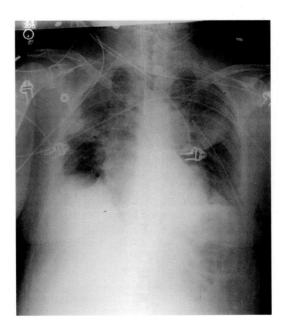

Answer: Optimization of COPD, lung expansion maneuvers, and postoperative pain control.

Discussion: COPD is the most important patient-related risk factor for postoperative pulmonary complications and increases risk by three to five fold. Physicians should prepare patients with COPD before surgery to minimize air flow obstruction, treat infection, and optimize functional status. Antibiotics are appropriate only for patients in whom a change in the character or amount of sputum suggests infection. There is no benefit of preoperative antibiotics in unselected patients with COPD. One should treat air flow obstruction in the same fashion as for patients not anticipating surgery. Combinations of chest physical therapy, inhaled bronchodilators, antibiotics, and corticosteroids have been shown to reduce the risk of postoperative pulmonary complications in high-risk patients. No studies have evaluated systematically, however, the benefit of individual agents.

All patients with clinically apparent COPD should receive inhaled ipratropium. Inhaled β-agonists are synergistic when added for symptomatic patients. Theophylline decreases dyspnea in patients who remain symptomatic despite the aforementioned therapies. Corticosteroids improve airway obstruction in approximately 20% of patients with COPD. If a patient with COPD is not at his or her best baseline before surgery, a 1- to 2-week course of systemic corticosteroids is appropriate unless he or she has been shown previously not to respond to such treatment. Patients who smoke should be encouraged to stop smoking for at least 8 weeks before surgery. This recommendation is based on the findings of two studies that showed an unexpected increase in risk for patients who had stopped smoking for less than 8 weeks before surgery.

When COPD is optimally treated, additional strategies reduce the risk of postoperative pulmonary complications in patients with COPD. When possible, limiting the duration of surgery to less than 3 hours, using spinal anesthesia, and avoiding pancuronium as a neuromuscular blocker are three intraoperative strategies to reduce risk. Pulmonary complication rates are significantly lower for laparoscopic abdominal procedures than for open abdominal surgeries and should be considered when possible.

After surgery, strategies to increase lung volumes and decrease pain reduce the incidence of postoperative pulmonary complications in high-risk patients. Deep breathing exercises and incentive spirometry each reduce this risk by one half. These strategies are more effective if first taught to patients before surgery rather than after surgery. Continuous positive airway pressure reduces risk similarly and may be used for patients who are unable to cooperate with the other lung expansion techniques. Epidural analgesia reduces risk in high-risk patients undergoing thoracic, abdominal, and major vascular surgeries. Studies of postoperative intercostal nerve blocks show more variable results, but there is a trend toward a similar reduction in risk.

The present patient is at high risk for pulmonary complications because of the history of poor exercise capacity, the physical findings of wheezing and a prolonged expiratory phase, and the high-risk thoracic and upper abdominal incisions. She would have had a lower risk of developing postoperative pneumonia if her physician systematically had applied the aforementioned risk reduction strategies.

Clinical Pearls

1. COPD is a major risk factor for postoperative pulmonary complications and increases risk by three to five fold.

2. Preoperative risk reduction strategies include instruction in lung expansion maneuvers, ipratropium, inhaled bronchodilators, antibiotics for patients with suspected bacterial respiratory infection, and systemic corticosteroids for patients whose air flow obstruction is not optimally minimized.

3. Intraoperative strategies include the use of spinal anesthesia, avoidance of pancuronium, limiting surgery to less than 3 hours when possible, and the use of laparoscopic abdominal procedures in lieu of open abdominal surgery.

4. Deep breathing exercises, incentive spirometry, continuous positive airway pressure, and epidural analgesia are effective postoperative strategies to reduce pulmonary complications in high-risk patients with COPD.

REFERENCES

1. Tarhan S, Moffitt EA, Sessler AD, et al: Risk of anesthesia and surgery in patients with chronic bronchitis and chronic obstructive pulmonary disease. Surgery 74:720–726, 1973.
2. Warner MA, Offord KP, Warner ME, et al: Role of preoperative cessation of smoking and other factors in postoperative pulmonary complications: A blinded prospective study of coronary artery bypass patients. Mayo Clin Proc 64:609–616, 1989.
3. Thomas JA, McIntosh JM: Are incentive spirometry, intermittent positive pressure breathing, and deep breathing exercises effective in the prevention of postoperative pulmonary complications after upper abdominal surgery? A systematic overview and meta-analysis. Phys Ther 74:3–16, 1994.
4. Brooks-Brunn JA: Postoperative atelectasis and pneumonia. Heart Lung 24:94–115, 1995.
5. Ballantyne JC, Carr DB, deFerranti S, et al: The comparative effects of postoperative analgesic therapies on pulmonary outcome: Cumulative meta-analyses of randomized, controlled trials. Anesth Analg 86:598–612, 1998.

PATIENT 10

A 34-year-old man with asthma scheduled for ventral hernia repair

A 34-year-old man presents to the preoperative testing area 1 week before elective repair of a ventral hernia. Ten years earlier, he had a midline laparotomy for repair of a perforated duodenal ulcer. He has a history of asthma dating to adolescence. He was last hospitalized for asthma 3 years ago and requires intermittent use of oral corticosteroids to control his symptoms; his last use of prednisone was 4 months ago. At baseline, he walks regularly for several miles without limitation. He recently has increased his use of an albuterol metered-dose inhaler to two to three times daily and is dyspneic with two flights of stairs. During the past 2 weeks, he has noted an increase in wheezing. He has a mild nonproductive cough. His baseline peak flow is 450. He is otherwise healthy without additional medical problems. Current medications include albuterol metered-dose inhaler, 2 puffs two to three times daily, and triamcinolone inhaler, 4 puffs twice daily.

Physical Examination: Temperature 98.4°F orally, heart rate 66, respirations 16, blood pressure 130/78. No respiratory distress at rest. HEENT: normal. Chest: mild decrease in breath sounds. Inspiratory-to-expiratory ratio of 1:2. Diffuse mild late expiratory wheezing. No focal rales or rhonchi. Cardiac: normal S_1 and S_2, no murmurs or gallops. Carotid upstrokes: normal. Abdomen: midline abdominal scar with large, easily reducible ventral hernia. Extremities: no edema.

Laboratory Findings: Hct 46%, WBC 6200/μL with normal differential. Peak flow 300. Chest radiograph: normal. ECG: see Figure next page.

Question: What is the risk of postoperative pulmonary complications in this patient?

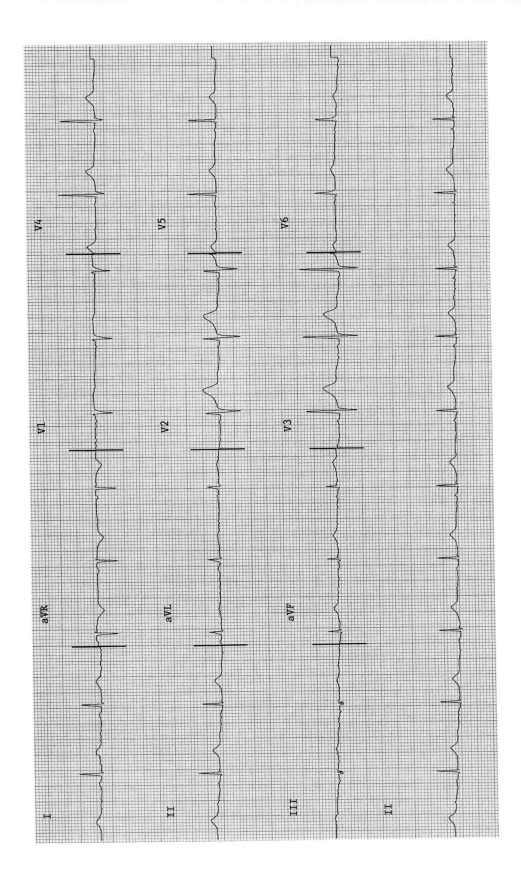

Answer: Well-controlled asthma is not an important risk factor for postoperative pulmonary complications.

Discussion: Asthma is a common chronic condition that affects more than 10 million Americans and accounts for 9 million physician office visits each year in the United States. Physicians often evaluate patients with asthma before surgery. Potential postoperative pulmonary complications include pneumonia, bronchitis, atelectasis, prolonged mechanical ventilation, and bronchospasm. Clinicians also must consider the perioperative management of patients with asthma who are or have been recently on systemic corticosteroids.

The risk of postoperative pulmonary complications among patients with asthma varies across studies but is consistently lower than the risk among patients with chronic obstructive pulmonary disease. In a large study of perioperative complications in patients with asthma, the overall incidence of complications was only 2%. Bronchospasm and laryngospasm were the most common complications. Of 706 patients, 2 developed postoperative respiratory failure, but there were no pneumonias or deaths in the entire sample. Other authors have reported similarly low complication rates among children with asthma undergoing surgery.

Although the overall perioperative complication rate for patients with asthma is low, certain surgery-specific factors increase the risk in this population. The surgical site is the most important additional risk factor; postoperative pulmonary complications are most common in thoracic and upper abdominal surgery. Pulmonary complications also are more common in surgeries lasting more than 3 hours and in patients receiving pancuronium as a neuromuscular blocking agent.

Historical features that suggest inadequate treatment of asthma include cough or wheeze with activity or at night, a change from the baseline pattern of cough or sputum, and the need for greater use of an inhaled β-agonist. Additional historical features help to classify severity of asthma and to predict the likelihood of admission for medical patients with asthma, including prior hospitalization for asthma, prior intubation for the treatment of asthma, recent or long-term systemic corticosteroid use, and frequent exacerbations or emergency department visits. In the previously mentioned series, these factors all predicted a higher risk of postoperative complications. The rate of postoperative laryngospasm or bronchospasm for patients with these features varied from 3% to 28%.

A peak flow should be measured in all patients with asthma preparing for surgery. A patient is in his or her optimal condition for surgery if the peak flow is greater than 80% of predicted or of the patient's personal best values. Routine preoperative chest radiographs are not helpful unless clinical features suggest infection.

Physicians should treat patients with asthma before surgery exactly as they would treat patients not preparing for surgery. Patients who are not at baseline by history or peak flow should be treated aggressively to reduce bronchospasm. Patients should continue inhaled β-agonists as needed for symptoms. These agents also may be used in the intraoperative and postoperative periods as needed for bronchospasm. Inhaled corticosteroids should be added or increased if air flow obstruction persists. Physicians should recommend antibiotics for patients with respiratory infection, but no evidence exists for their indiscriminate use before surgery.

Clinicians often worry about the use of preoperative systemic corticosteroids because of concern for potentially increasing the risk of perioperative infection. Investigators have evaluated the risk of pulmonary, wound, and all perioperative infections among steroid-dependent asthmatics and those who received a 1-week course of preoperative high-dose systemic corticosteroids to optimize their condition. In both cases, no difference existed in the low rate of perioperative infections between corticosteroid-treated patients and control patients not receiving systemic corticosteroids. It is safe to use a 1- to 2-week preoperative course of oral corticosteroids to decrease air flow obstruction in asthmatic patients who are not in their optimal condition despite other treatments.

In the present patient, the ECG is normal, but the history establishes that he is not at his personal best baseline. His symptoms and need for inhaled bronchodilators have increased, his exercise capacity is diminished, and his peak flow is reduced to 67% of baseline. He should be treated with oral corticosteroids for 1 to 2 weeks to render him free of wheezes and to achieve a peak flow of greater than 80% of his baseline.

Clinical Pearls

1. Well-controlled asthma is a minimal risk factor for postoperative pulmonary complications.

2. Upper abdominal and thoracic surgeries confer the greatest risk of postoperative pulmonary complications in patients with asthma.

3. Patients with asthma should be treated before surgery until they are free of wheezes and have a peak flow of at least 80% of predicted or of their personal best.

4. Preoperative systemic corticosteroids may be used safely without increasing the risk of infection for patients whose air flow obstruction is not reduced optimally by other therapies.

REFERENCES

1. Gold MI, Helrich M: A study of complications related to anesthesia in asthmatic patients. Anesth Analg 42:283–293, 1963.
2. Pien LC, Grammer LC, Patterson R: Minimal complications in a surgical population with severe asthma receiving prophylactic corticosteroids. J Allergy Clin Immunol 82:696–700, 1988.
3. Guidelines for the diagnosis and management of asthma. National Heart, Lung, and Blood Institute, National Asthma Education Program, expert panel report. X. Special considerations. J Allergy Clin Immunol 88(suppl):523–534, 1991.
4. Kabalin CS, Yarnold PR, Grammer LC: Low complication rate of corticosteroid-treated asthmatics undergoing surgical procedures. Arch Intern Med 155:1379–1384, 1995.
5. Warner DO, Warner MA, Barnes RD, et al: Perioperative respiratory complications in patients with asthma. Anesthesiology 85:460–467, 1996.

PATIENT 11

A 53-year-old woman scheduled for laparoscopic cholecystectomy

A 53-year-old woman has had four episodes of biliary pain over the past 6 months, each characterized by 3 to 4 hours of right upper quadrant pain and nausea. Abdominal ultrasound confirmed the presence of gallstones. She now is scheduled for elective laparoscopic cholecystectomy and awaits evaluation in the preoperative testing center. Her past medical history is notable only for hypertension and migraine headaches. Her only regular medication is atenolol.

Physical Examination: Temperature 98.4°F, blood pressure 144/86, heart rate 56, respirations 12. General appearance: well, but obese. Chest: clear to auscultation and percussion. Cardiac: normal S_1S_2 without murmurs, gallops, or rub. Abdomen: obese, soft, and nontender. No hepatosplenomegaly or masses. Extremities: no edema.

Laboratory Findings: Hct 38%, WBC 5400/μL. ALT 36, AST 30, alkaline phosphatase 86, total bilirubin 1.1. Chest radiograph normal. ECG (see next page): left ventricular hypertrophy.

Questions: What is the perioperative cardiac and pulmonary risk for this patient undergoing laparoscopic cholecystectomy? How does this risk differ from that of a traditional open cholecystectomy?

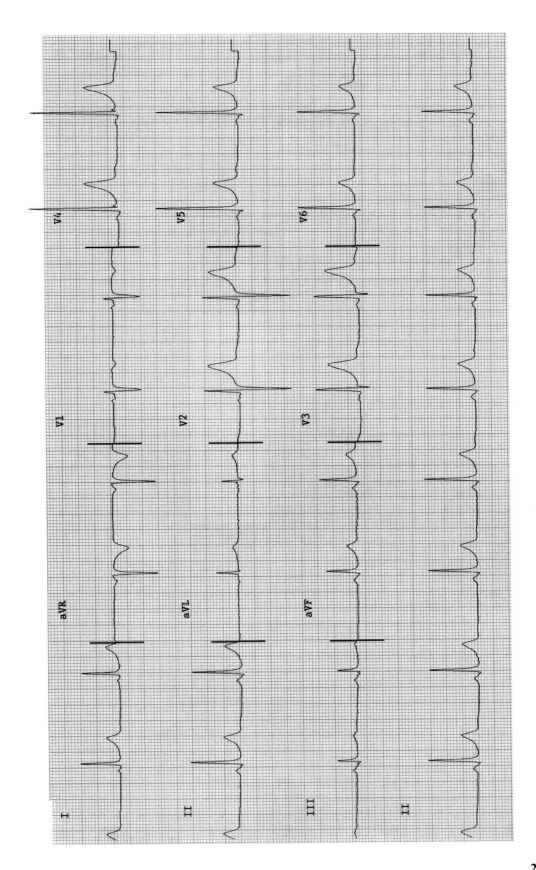

Answer: Laparoscopic cholecystectomy has a low incidence of postoperative pulmonary complications, but an incidence of cardiac complications that is similar to open cholecystectomy.

Discussion: Laparoscopic cholecystectomy first was introduced in the United States in 1988. Since then, this technique became the standard surgical approach to the management of symptomatic gallstones and now accounts for >90% of cholecystectomies. The abdomen is insufflated with carbon dioxide to maintain a pneumoperitoneum. Four incisions are made in the abdomen to introduce the laparoscope and surgical instruments. Patients undergoing laparoscopic cholecystectomy receive general anesthesia because of patient discomfort associated with the creation of a pneumoperitoneum.

As a result of the rapid acceptance of this procedure by the medical community, few controlled trials exist that compare laparoscopic with open cholecystectomy. In a 1994 British trial, investigators randomized 302 patients with symptomatic gallstones to one or the other procedure. Intraoperative time was 14 minutes longer in the laparoscopic group, although overall hospital stay was shorter by 2 days. There was no difference in any surgical complication or total complications between the two groups. Pulmonary infection (not further characterized) occurred in one patient undergoing laparoscopic surgery and five patients undergoing minilaparotomy. Patients in the laparoscopic group returned to leisure activities sooner, but there was no difference in the time to return to employment between the two groups.

Other studies have found less postoperative pain, shorter hospital stays, greater patient satisfaction with the appearance of the scars, and more rapid return to full activities and employment among patients undergoing laparoscopic cholecystectomy. In 2% to 5% of cases, surgical findings necessitate the conversion of an intended laparoscopic procedure to open cholecystectomy. Physicians should not recommend laparoscopic cholecystectomy to patients whom they believe to be at unacceptable risk for an open procedure because this conversion may be necessary.

The mortality of laparoscopic cholecystectomy is lower than that of open cholecystectomy and ranges from 0 to 1% in large published series (see Table). Pulmonary complications are common after open upper abdominal surgery. They are substantially less common with laparoscopic cholecystectomy. Pneumonia and atelectasis were significantly less common in laparoscopic procedures in a study comparing the prelaparoscopic and postlaparoscopic eras. Pneumonia occurred in 2.3% of open procedures and 0.5% of laparoscopic procedures; atelectasis occurred in 10% and 5.4%. The lower rate of postoperative pulmonary complications is one of the most compelling advantages of laparoscopic cholecystectomy and supports its use in patients who are at high risk for pulmonary complications.

Patients with chronic obstructive pulmonary disease have a greater likelihood of developing intraoperative hypercarbia resulting from carbon dioxide insufflation than do healthy patients. Preoperative hypercarbia does not increase this risk incrementally, however. No data suggest that intraoperative hypercarbia increases the risk of clinically significant postoperative pulmonary complications, although refractory acidosis occasionally may necessitate conversion to an open cholecystectomy.

Fewer studies have evaluated cardiac complications, but available data suggest similar rates of postoperative cardiac complications between the two procedures; this may reflect the comparable anesthetic technique and duration of surgery be-

Comparison of Rates of Mortality and Selected Medical Complications
in Laparoscopic Versus Open Cholecystectomy

Study	No. Patients		Death (%)		Pneumonia (%)		Atelectasis (%)		MI (%)	
	Lap	Open	Lap	Open	Lap	Open	Lap	Open	Lap	Open
Chen, 1998	1300	2018	0.2	1.6						
Shea, 1998	1611	2031	0.4	1.5	0.5	2.3	5.4	10.0	0.1	0.1
Hall, 1996	37	58	0	0	0	0	3	17		
McMahon, 1994	151	148	0	0.7	0.7	3.4			0	0.7
Steiner, 1994	14,274	15,577	0.15	1.6						
Schauer, 1993	20	20	0	0	0	5	5	35		

Lap = Laparoscopic cholecystectomy, Open = open cholecystectomy, MI = myocardial infarction.

tween the two procedures. Several small case series have reported acceptable risks of postoperative cardiac events in patients who were at high risk secondary to preexisting cardiac disease and high American Society of Anesthesiologists (ASA) class. In a study of 13 laparoscopic biliary procedures among patients with cardiac disease and an ASA class of III or IV, one patient developed a supraventricular arrhythmia that responded to treatment, and there was one death in a patient with significant aortic stenosis. The other patients had an uneventful postoperative course.

In the present case, the patient had no factors that would increase her risk above procedure-specific baselines for postoperative cardiac or pulmonary complications. She could proceed to surgery with a low overall risk of cardiac and pulmonary complications and mortality.

Clinical Pearls

1. Laparoscopic cholecystectomy carries a lower operative mortality than traditional, open cholecystectomy.

2. Patients undergoing laparoscopic cholecystectomy require general anesthesia.

3. Postoperative pulmonary complications are significantly less common in laparoscopic cholecystectomy than in open cholecystectomy.

4. Patients undergoing laparoscopic cholecystectomy have less postoperative pain, shorter hospital stays, and a more rapid return to full activities than patients undergoing open cholecystectomy.

REFERENCES

1. Carroll BJ, Chandra M, Phillips EH, Margulies DR: Laparoscopic cholecystectomy in critically ill cardiac patients. Am Surg 59:783–785, 1993.
2. Wittgen CM, Naunheim KS, Andrus CH, et al: Preoperative pulmonary function evaluation for laparoscopic cholecystectomy. Arch Surg 128:880–886, 1993.
3. McMahon AJ, Russell IT, Baxter JN, et al: Laparoscopic verus minilaparotomy cholecystectomy: A randomised trial. Lancet 343:135–138, 1994.
4. Steiner CA, Bass EB, Talamini MA, et al: Surgical rates and operative mortality for open and laparoscopic cholecystectomy in Maryland. N Engl J Med 330:403–408, 1994.
5. Chen AY, Daley J, Pappas TN, et al: Growing use of laparoscopic cholecystectomy in the National Veterans Affairs Surgical Risk Study: Effects on volume, patient selection, and selected outcomes. Ann Surg 227:12–24, 1998.
6. Shea JA, Berlin JA, Bachwich DR, et al: Indications for and outcomes of cholecystectomy: A comparison of the pre and post-laparoscopic eras. Ann Surg 227:343–350, 1998.

PATIENT 12

A 64-year-old man with coronary artery disease
scheduled for elective hemicolectomy

A 64-year-old man is scheduled for an elective right hemicolectomy for adenocarcinoma. He has a 3-year history of stable exertional angina. An exercise tolerance test 2 years ago showed 2-mm ST depression in the inferior leads at 8 minutes into a standard Bruce protocol with a rate pressure product of 26,000. He now experiences angina ascending three flights of stairs or jogging >15 minutes. He has no pain at rest or with walking. There has been no recent change in his symptoms. Past medical history also includes hypertension and hypercholesterolemia. Medications include aspirin, isosorbide mononitrate, amlodipine, and sublingual nitroglycerin on an as-needed basis.

Physical Examination: Blood pressure 130/84, heart rate 66, respirations 14. General appearance: a well-appearing man in no distress. Chest: clear to auscultation and percussion. Cardiac: regular rhythm, normal S_1 and S_2, soft S_4. No murmurs or rubs. Extremities: no edema.

Laboratory Findings: Hct 44%, WBC 7200/μL. ECG: normal.

Question: How can the risk of perioperative cardiac complications be reduced in this patient with coronary artery disease (CAD)?

Answer: Use perioperative β-blockers to reduce cardiac risk.

Discussion: Postoperative cardiac complications are the major source of surgical morbidity other than complications related to the surgical condition itself. An important risk factor for the development of cardiac complications is the presence of known CAD. Published cardiac risk indices differ on the importance of stable angina as a risk factor. In Goldman's original cardiac risk index, stable angina was not a risk factor for postoperative cardiac complications. In the revised cardiac risk index, current stable angina was a risk factor. When evaluating patients with known CAD before surgery, several strategies exist to reduce the risk of cardiac complications.

The most important intervention to reduce risk is the use of perioperative β-blockers. Two large randomized controlled trials have shown the benefit of perioperative β-blockers in selected patients. In the first, Mangano et al studied 200 patients undergoing elective surgery who had either known CAD (previous myocardial infarction, typical angina, or atypical angina with a positive stress test) or two risk factors for CAD (age >65 years, hypertension, smoking, serum cholesterol ≥240 mg/dL, and diabetes). Study patients received intravenous atenolol 30 minutes before surgery, immediately after surgery, and every 12 hours after surgery until taking oral medications. When taking oral medications, patients received oral atenolol until hospital discharge up to a maximum of 7 days. The results were striking. One-year mortality was 3% in the atenolol group and 14% in the placebo group. The American College of Physicians has recommended the use of atenolol in this fashion for all patients who meet the eligibility criteria of this study.

Another study evaluated the benefit of oral bisoprolol for high-risk patients undergoing major vascular surgery. In this study, all patients were at high risk because of an abnormal dobutamine echocardiogram and at least one additional risk factor. Treated patients received oral bisoprolol for 1 week before surgery and continued until 30 days after surgery. The combined end point of cardiac death or nonfatal myocardial infarction occurred in 3% of the bisoprolol group and 34% of the placebo group. These results were similar to those of the atenolol study.

No randomized controlled trials exist of the value of coronary revascularization as a strategy to reduce the risk of subsequent noncardiac surgery. Retrospective data of patients undergoing coronary artery bypass graft (CABG) surgery and percutaneous transluminal coronary angioplasty (PTCA) have shown only modest risk reduction. In a retrospective analysis of the Coronary Artery Surgery Study (CASS) database, the reduction in mortality for high-risk noncardiac surgery among patients with CAD previously randomized to CABG surgery (versus medical therapy) was similar to the risk of the CABG surgery itself.

An uncontrolled retrospective study evaluated the risk of perioperative cardiac complications among patients with CAD who had been treated medically or by PTCA. Rates of angina and congestive heart failure were lower in the PTCA-treated group, but no difference existed in the rates of cardiac death (2% to 3%) or myocardial infarction (3%) between the two groups. The American College of Physicians and American College of Cardiology guidelines recommend revascularization as a risk reduction strategy only if the patient has an indication separate from the need for noncardiac surgery.

The present patient meets the criteria for perioperative β-blockers according to the study of Mangano et al and the American College of Physicians guideline. Even if he were taking long-term β-blockers, he should receive intravenous β-blockers in the perioperative period to keep the heart rate <80 beats/min until he is able to take oral β-blockers postoperatively.

Clinical Pearls

1. Use perioperative β-blockers for patients with CAD or at least two risk factors for CAD, unless a compelling contraindication exists.

2. Use intravenous β-blockers for such patients in the immediate perioperative period while unable to take oral mediations. This recommendation also applies to patients who were taking long-term β-blockers before surgery.

3. Current data do not support coronary revascularization as a strategy to reduce the risk of noncardiac surgery, unless the patient has an indication for revascularization separate from the need for noncardiac surgery.

REFERENCES

1. Goldman L, Caldera DL, Nussbaum SR, et al: Multifactorial index of cardiac risk in noncardiac surgical procedures. N Engl J Med 297:845–850, 1977.
2. Mangano DT, Layug EL, Wallace A, et al: Effect of atenolol on mortality and cardiovascular morbidity after noncardiac surgery. N Engl J Med 335:1713–1720, 1996.
3. Eagle KA, Rihal CS, Mickel MC, et al: Cardiac risk of noncardiac surgery: Influence of coronary disease and type of surgery in 3369 operations. Circulation 96:1882–1887, 1997.
4. Lee TH, Marcantonio ER, Mangione CM, et al: Derivation and prospective validation of a simple index for prediction of cardiac risk of major noncardiac surgery. Circulation 100:1043–1049, 1999.
5. Poldermans D, Boersma E, Bax JJ, et al: The effect of bisoprolol on perioperative mortality and myocardial infarction in high-risk patients undergoing vascular surgery. N Engl J Med 341:1789–1794, 1999.
6. Posner KL, Van Norman GA, Chan V: Adverse cardiac outcomes after noncardiac surgery in patients with prior percutaneous transluminal coronary angioplasty. Anesth Analg 89:553–560, 1999.

PATIENT 13

A 53-year-old man with hypertension preparing for elective cervical laminectomy

A 53 year-old man has a history of unremitting pain in his neck radiating to his right arm associated with right hand weakness. Magnetic resonance imaging confirmed a large C5–C6 central disc herniation with canal stenosis and cord impingement. He is now scheduled for a cervical laminectomy and discectomy. Past medical history includes hypertension but is otherwise negative. Medications are atenolol 50 mg daily, and hydrochlorothiazide 25 mg daily.

Physical Examination: Temperature 98.6°F, blood pressure 160/102, heart rate 56, respiratory rate 12. HEENT: normal except for mild hypertensive arteriolar narrowing on funduscopic exam. Chest: clear. Cardiac: normal S1, S2 with an S4. No S3, murmur, or rub. Jugular venous pressure is normal. Extremities: no edema.

Laboratory Findings: CBC: normal, Na 142, K 3.6, Cl 107, CO2 24, BUN 12, creatinine 0.8. Electrocardiogram (see next page): left ventricular hypertrophy; otherwise normal.

Questions: Is hypertension a risk factor for postoperative cardiac complications? Should surgery be delayed?

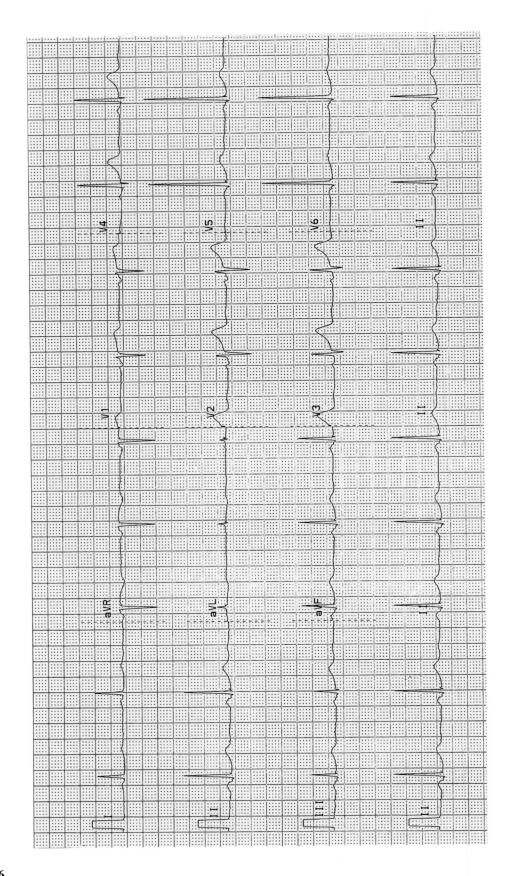

Answer: Mild to moderate hypertension is not a risk factor for postoperative cardiac complications. Surgery need not be delayed for hypertension unless the diastolic blood pressure is > 110.

Discussion: Hypertension accounts for more physician office visits than any other chronic illness and is present in approximately 25 percent of the adult population. While hypertension is a major risk factor for the development of stroke and coronary artery disease, most studies have not found mild to moderate hypertension to be an independent risk factor for the development of postoperative cardiac complications. In an early large study, Goldman and Caldera studied the cardiac outcomes of surgery among 676 patients, 196 of whom were hypertensive. Patients with hypertension and diastolic blood pressure < 110 had higher rates of perioperative hypertension but no increase in the risk of postoperative cardiac complications.

The risk of more severe hypertension with preoperative diastolic blood pressures > 110 is less well studied. Early studies suggest both an increased risk of intraoperative blood pressure lability and clinically important cardiac complications. Physicians should delay elective surgery if diastolic blood pressure is > 110 in order to effectively treat and reduce the blood pressure.

Three validated multifactorial risk indices (Goldman, Detsky, Lee; see references Case 14) now exist for the prediction of postoperative cardiac complications. None of these indices identified hypertension as a predictor in their multivariate analyses. Two consensus guidelines for perioperative cardiac evaluation have proposed hypertension as a minor risk factor. In the American College of Physicians guideline, hypertension is not one of the principle factors used to estimate risk. It is one of several factors used to determine the need for pharmacologic stress testing for patients undergoing vascular surgery but does not appear in the stratification algorithm for patients undergoing non-vascular surgery. In the contemporaneous American College of Cardiology/American Heart Association guideline, uncontrolled systemic hypertension is considered a minor clinical predictor that does not influence decision making related to risk assessment.

While surgery need not be delayed for a patient with stable hypertension and a diastolic blood pressure <110, if time is available before surgery, medications should be adjusted to achieve a more desirable blood pressure of <140/90. In general, antihypertensive therapy should be continued through the morning of surgery and may be given with sips of water on the morning of the procedure. Concerns related to blunting of intraoperative hemodynamic responses and response to pharmacologic intervention in the operating room have proven unfounded. Rather, abrupt discontinuation of antihypertensive therapy before surgery may lead to rebound hypertension and increased blood pressure lability in the perioperative period.

The risk of rebound hypertension is greatest for patients who are taking beta-blockers or clonidine. In fact, continuation of beta-blockers throughout the perioperative period reduces the risk of postoperative cardiac complications among patients with coronary artery disease or at least two risk factors for coronary disease (including age ≥ 65, hypertension, cigarette use, cholesterol ≥ 240, and diabetes). This was shown in a study of normotensive and hypertensive patients undergoing noncardiac surgery. These data suggest that hypertensive patients who are not currently taking beta-blockers, and who meet the above criteria, should be treated with perioperative beta-blockers in order to reduce the risk of postoperative cardiac complications. No other class of antihypertensive agents has been specifically shown to reduce the risk of cardiac complications of surgery.

Patients taking diuretics for the treatment of hypertension are at risk for volume depletion and hypokalemia. These patients should have a routine measurement of the serum potassium level before elective surgery and any abnormalities should be corrected. Clinically important volume depletion is uncommon in patients who are chronically on a stable dose of a thiazide diuretic; however clinicians should estimate volume status on such patients before surgery. Some authors suggest holding diuretics for two days before surgery; the advantages of this approach are unknown. Likewise, the use of angiotensin-converting enzyme (ACE) inhibitors before surgery may blunt compensatory responses during surgery and increase the risk of perioperative hypotension. Intraoperative hypotension due to ACE inhibitors responds to ephedrine. Given the risk of poorly controlled hypertension if these medications are withdrawn before surgery, it is reasonable to continue them through the morning of surgery although further study and consensus is needed on this point.

In the present case, blood pressure is above conventionally accepted goals for the prevention of long-term complications but is below the range associated with an increased risk of postoperative complications. Surgery need not be delayed for this blood pressure reading; however if time exists, medications may be adjusted to achieve an optimal blood pressure of <140/90. He should have a measurement of serum potassium before surgery and a clinical estimation of volume status on the day of surgery. The patient should receive his beta-blocker throughout the perioperative period including an oral dose on the morning of surgery and parenteral beta-blockers as necessary in the operating room and immediately after surgery to maintain blood pressure and heart rate at acceptable values.

Clinical Pearls

1. Mild to moderate hypertension is not a risk factor for postoperative cardiac complications.

2. A diastolic blood pressure of >110 increases the risk of postoperative cardiac complications; elective surgery should be delayed until this is treated.

3. All antihypertensive medications, with the possible exception of diuretics and ACE inhibitors, should be continued through the morning of surgery.

4. Among antihypertensive agents, only beta-blockers have been specifically shown to reduce the risk of cardiac complications in a subset of patients with coronary artery disease, or at least two risk factors for coronary artery disease.

REFERENCES

1. Goldman L, Caldera DL. Risks of general anesthesia and elective operation in the hypertensive patient. Anesthesiology 50:285–292, 1979.
2. Wolsthal SD. Is blood pressure control necessary before surgery? Med Clin N Amer 77:349–363, 1993.
3. American College of Cardiology/American Heart Association task force on practice guidelines (committee on perioperative cardiovascular evaluation for noncardiac surgery). Guidelines for perioperative cardiovascular evaluation for noncardiac surgery. Circulation 93:1278–1317, 1996.
4. Mangano DT, Layug EL, Wallace A, et al: Effect of atenolol on mortality and cardiovascular morbidity after noncardiac surgery. N Engl J Med 335;1713–1720, 1996.
5. Smith MS, Muir H, Hall R. Perioperative management of drug therapy: clinical considerations. Drugs 51:238–259, 1996.
6. American College of Physicians. Guidelines for assessing and managing the perioperative risk from coronary artery disease associated with major noncardiac surgery. Ann Intern Med 127:309–312, 1997.

PATIENT 14

An 80-year-old man with aortic stenosis scheduled for transurethral resection of the prostate

An 80-year-old man with a long history of prostatism symptoms has nocturia three times each night and difficulty initiating his urinary stream. After failing to respond to medication, he now is scheduled for an elective transurethral resection of the prostate. Medical history includes hypertension, a remote history of cholecystectomy, and moderately severe aortic stenosis. He has no history of angina, syncope, or congestive heart failure. He takes antibiotic prophylaxis for dental procedures. Medications include aspirin, nifedipine, and hydrochlorothiazide.

Physical Examination: Temperature 37°C, blood pressure 160/72, heart rate 72, respirations 14. HEENT: normal. Chest: clear. Cardiac: Regular rhythm. Hyperdynamic point of maximal impulse at apex. Normal S_1 with single soft S_2, III/VI harsh late peaking systolic ejection murmur at left upper sternal border. Carotid upstrokes are delayed.

Laboratory Findings: CBC, electrolytes, BUN, and creatinine all normal. ECG: normal sinus rhythm at 70, left-axis deviation, left ventricular hypertrophy with strain pattern, no Q waves. Transthoracic echocardiogram (long-axis view, *top*; short-axis view, *bottom*): moderately severe aortic stenosis with a thickened, deformed aortic valve (area 0.8 cm^2) (see Figures).

Question: What is the surgical risk associated with this patient's aortic stenosis?

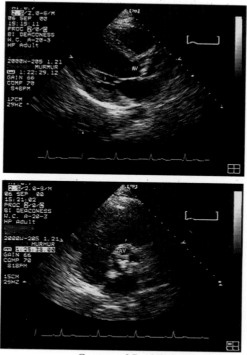

Courtesy of Carol Waksmonski, M.D.

Answer: Aortic stenosis poses a mild increase in the risk of postoperative cardiac complications.

Discussion: Goldman et al first identified significant aortic stenosis as a risk factor for postoperative cardiac complications in their landmark cardiac risk index published in 1977. They defined aortic stenosis broadly to include an ejection murmur of at least II/VI associated with compatible carotid and cardiac examinations or confirmation by diagnostic testing. These authors did not ascertain symptoms attributed to aortic stenosis. In the multivariate analysis, aortic stenosis was a minor risk factor and was assigned only 3 points out of a total of 53 points; this compared, for example, with 11 points for an S_3 gallop.

Subsequent studies and risk indices have varied in the importance assigned to aortic stenosis in estimating the risk of cardiac complications. Detsky et al developed a modified cardiac risk index that assigned 20 points to suspected critical aortic stenosis, defined as suspected 50 mmHg gradient based on symptoms, characteristic physical examination, and left ventricular hypertrophy on physical examination. This index performed equally well as the original Goldman index and forms the basis for the initial risk stratification in the American College of Physicians guideline for the assessment of perioperative cardiac risk. In the most recent index, the revised cardiac risk index, significant valvular heart disease conferred a relative risk of 3.2 for postoperative cardiac complications, but the factor was not significant in the logistic regression analysis and does not appear in the final risk index.

Several studies evaluated the risk of noncardiac surgery directly among patients with aortic stenosis. These studies suggested that the risk of aortic stenosis is modest, even among patients with severe or critical aortic stenosis. O'Keefe et al reported only five adverse cardiac events among 23 patients with significant aortic stenosis; there were no sequelae and no cardiac deaths. In a case-control study, patients with aortic stenosis were matched to similar patients without aortic stenosis. There was no difference in the rates of postoperative cardiac complications.

In another study, authors evaluated the risk of noncardiac surgery among patients with severe aortic stenosis undergoing 28 procedures. These patients all had a valve area of ≤ 0.5 cm^2 (i.e., critical aortic stenosis) and either refused or were not candidates for aortic valve replacement. Two patients died, and there were no other postoperative cardiac complications. This perioperative mortality is modest and suggests that lifesaving or other urgent surgery need not be denied to patients with critical aortic stenosis.

No data exist to determine the risk of noncardiac surgery among patients with aortic insufficiency. In the absence of specific data, it is reasonable to approach risk estimation for these patients as one would for patients with congestive heart failure. In a patient with aortic insufficiency who is well compensated with good exercise capacity, normal ventricular dimensions, and no congestive heart failure, the risk of surgery is average. In a patient with congestive heart failure, clinicians may estimate risk in the same fashion as any other patient with heart failure. Using the Goldman risk index, the findings of jugular venous distention or an S_3 each would increase risk. Patients with any significant aortic valvular disease also would require antibiotic prophylaxis as dictated by the type of surgery and the American Heart Association guidelines.

In the present case, the patient had moderately severe, but not critical, aortic stenosis. He had fair exercise capacity and no evidence of congestive heart failure. His risk for postoperative cardiac complications was mildly increased over baseline. Because he had no other symptomatic indications for aortic valve replacement, the morbidity and mortality of sequential aortic valve surgery followed by prostate surgery were not justified. If he and his primary care physician believed that the severity of symptoms from prostatism was unacceptable, he could proceed to surgery with a mild increase in risk. He would need antibiotic prophylaxis.

Clinical Pearls

1. Aortic stenosis is a risk factor for postoperative cardiac complications.
2. The magnitude of the risk varies according to differing risk indices.
3. Patients with severe or critical aortic stenosis can undergo surgery with an acceptable degree of risk if the indication for surgery is sufficiently compelling.

REFERENCES

1. Goldman L, Caldera DL, Nussbaum SR, et al: Multifactorial index of cardiac risk in noncardiac surgical procedures. N Engl J Med 297:845–850, 1977.
2. Detsky AS, Abrams HB, McLaughlin JR, et al: Predicting cardiac complications in patients undergoing non-cardiac surgery. J Gen Intern Med 1:211–219, 1986.
3. O'Keefe JH, Shub C, Rettke SR: Risk of noncardiac surgical procedures in patients with aortic stenosis. Mayo Clin Proc 64:400–405, 1989.
4. Raymer K, Yang H: Patients with aortic stenosis: Cardiac complications in non-cardiac surgery. Can J Anaesth 45:855–869, 1998.
5. Torsher LC, Shub C, Rettke SR, Brown DL: Risk of patients with severe aortic stenosis undergoing noncardiac surgery. Am J Cardiol 81:448–452, 1998.
6. Lee TH, Marcantonio ER, Mangione CM, et al: Derivation and prospective validation of a simple index for prediction of cardiac risk of major noncardiac surgery. Circulation 100:1043–1049, 1999.

PATIENT 15

A 63-year-old woman with mitral regurgitation scheduled for elective abdominal hysterectomy

A 63-year-old postmenopausal woman is scheduled for an elective abdominal hysterectomy for early-stage endometrial cancer. She is referred for preoperative medical evaluation because of a history of mitral regurgitation. She has had known mitral regurgitation for 5 years, which first was detected on routine physical examination. Her most recent echocardiogram 3 years ago showed moderate-to-severe mitral regurgitation with preserved left ventricular function and normal left ventricular end-diastolic dimensions. At baseline, she can walk 2 miles before resting because of knee pain. There is no history of exertional dyspnea. She is otherwise in good health. Medications include lisinopril, 20 mg daily, and aspirin, 325 mg daily.

Physical Examination: Blood pressure 130/76, heart rate 72, respiratory rate 14. Chest: clear. Cardiac: normal S_1S_2 with no S3 or S4. III/VI holosystolic murmur heard best at the apex with radiation across precordium. Normal left ventricular impulse. Carotid upstrokes brisk, jugular venous pressure 6 cm. Extremities: no edema.

Laboratory Findings: CBC, electrolytes, BUN, and creatinine all normal. Chest radiograph: left ventricular prominence but otherwise normal. ECG normal.

Question: What is the perioperative risk associated with mitral regurgitation?

Answer: Mitral regurgitation is not an independent risk factor for postoperative cardiac complications in the absence of congestive heart failure.

Discussion: The most common reason for requests for preoperative medical evaluation is to determine the risk of postoperative cardiac complications. Significant aortic stenosis is a mild risk factor for postoperative cardiac complications. Less is known about the risk associated with mitral valvular disease. The severity of mitral stenosis may be difficult to determine by physical examination alone. Likewise, it is not possible to determine the presence of early left ventricular dilation or decompensation in patients with mitral regurgitation by physical examination. Patients with suspected significant mitral valvular disease benefit from a preoperative echocardiogram to assess severity and guide management, unless a study has been obtained recently.

Neither mitral regurgitation nor mitral stenosis is an independent risk factor for cardiac complications in any of the published cardiac risk indices. In Goldman et al's original data, mitral regurgitation, but not mitral stenosis, was a univariate predictor of postoperative cardiac complications. In the multivariate analysis, mitral regurgitation did not hold up as a risk factor and does not appear in the Goldman cardiac risk index. The revised cardiac risk index and the guideline of the American College of Physicians do not include mitral regurgitation as a significant risk factor. The American College of Cardiology and American Heart Association guideline is ambiguous with regard to the risk of mitral valvular disease. In their guideline, severe valvular disease is considered to be a major clinical predictor of postoperative events. The text of the guideline principally identifies severe aortic stenosis as a risk factor, however, and provides no primary data to support mitral regurgitation as a risk factor. No studies have evaluated specifically the perioperative cardiac risk attributed to mitral valvular disease.

Congestive heart failure is a major risk factor for postoperative cardiac complications. Goldman et al first identified the presence of an S_3 or jugular venous distention as significant predictors. In the revised cardiac risk index, any of the following indicators of congestive heart failure predicted risk: a history of congestive heart failure, pulmonary edema, paroxysmal nocturnal dyspnea, bilateral rales or S_3 gallop, or a chest radiograph showing pulmonary vascular redistribution. A patient with poorly compensated mitral valvular disease who has any of these findings has an increased risk of postoperative cardiac complications.

Physicians should treat patients with significant mitral valve disease who are preparing for noncardiac surgery in exactly the same fashion as patients not anticipating surgery. Patients who have an independent indication for valve repair or replacement are candidates for such surgery, but physicians should not recommend surgical management of mitral valve disease to reduce the risk of noncardiac surgery, unless one of these independent indications is present. Afterload reduction with an angiotensin-converting enzyme inhibitor is appropriate for patients with significant mitral regurgitation; diuretics are used in the usual fashion for symptomatic pulmonary congestion.

For patients with mitral stenosis, heart rate control is important in the perioperative period to minimize perioperative pulmonary edema resulting from tachycardia and decreased diastolic filling time; perioperative β-blockers should be used to treat rapid ventricular rates for patients in sinus rhythm and patients in atrial fibrillation. For patients with moderate or severe mitral stenosis undergoing major surgery, right heart catheterization should be considered.

All patients with significant valvular heart disease should receive antibiotic prophylaxis according to the American Heart Association criteria.

In the present case, the patient had good exercise capacity and no evidence of congestive heart failure or decreased cardiac reserve by history or physical examination. An echocardiogram 3 years ago showed normal left ventricular function and dimensions. The echocardiogram should be repeated before her elective surgery to confirm that there had been no change in left ventricular function. If the echocardiogram was unchanged, she could proceed to surgery with no increase in the risk of postoperative cardiac complications.

Clinical Pearls

1. Neither mitral stenosis nor mitral regurgitation is an independent risk factor for the development of postoperative cardiac complications or for perioperative cardiac death.

2. The indications for surgery for mitral valve disease are the same for patients preparing for noncardiac surgery as for patients who are not anticipating surgery.

3. Patients with mitral stenosis are particularly sensitive to the effects of tachycardia, and heart rate should be controlled with perioperative β-blockers.

4. Perioperative right heart catheterization should be considered to guide fluid management for patients with significant mitral stenosis.

5. Antibiotics for endocarditis prophylaxis should be used as indicated by the American Heart Association criteria.

REFERENCES

1. Goldman L, Caldera DL, Nussbaum SR, et al: Multifactorial index of cardiac risk in noncardiac surgical procedures. N Engl J Med 297:845–850, 1977.
2. American College of Cardiology/American Heart Association task force on practice guidelines: Guidelines for perioperative cardiovascular evaluation for noncardiac surgery. Circulation 93:1278–1317, 1996.
3. Lee TH, Marcantonio ER, Mangione CM, et al: Derivation and prospective validation of a simple index for prediction of cardiac risk of major noncardiac surgery. Circulation 100:1043–1049, 1999.

PATIENT 16

An 83-year-old man presenting for preoperative medical evaluation before elective cataract surgery

An 83-year-old man has a 3-year history of progressive decrease in vision in the left eye. He is scheduled for elective cataract surgery and referred to the preoperative testing center for medical evaluation. Past medical history includes stable angina that occurs at three blocks walking on level ground, hypertension, and hypercholesterolemia. He had an uneventful repair of an inguinal hernia under general anesthesia 5 years ago. Medications are atenolol, 50 mg daily; aspirin, 325 mg daily; and atorvastatin, 10 mg daily. He has no known drug allergies.

Physical Examination: Blood pressure 140/82, heart rate 56, respirations 12. Chest: clear to auscultation and percussion. Cardiac: normal S_1 and S_2; S_4 is present. No murmurs. Carotid upstrokes normal.

Laboratory Findings: CBC: normal. SMA-7: normal. ECG: left ventricular hypertrophy, otherwise normal. Chest radiograph: normal. Slit-lamp examination: mature nuclear cataract (see Figure).

Questions: What is the optimal preoperative evaluation for this patient? Does routine laboratory testing incrementally modify preoperative risk assessment?

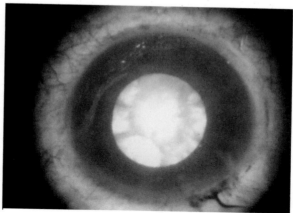

Courtesy of Mark Kuperwaser, M.D.

Answers: Cataract surgery is a low-risk surgery under conscious sedation. Laboratory testing does not have a substantial impact on patient selection, risk assessment, or management.

Discussion: Cataract surgery is the most commonly performed surgical procedure among elderly people in the United States and is a frequent reason for preoperative medical consultation. More than 1.5 million cataract surgeries are performed each year in the United States. Physicians performing preoperative assessments should be familiar with the risks of this surgery and the value of preoperative evaluation and testing. Overall morbidity resulting from cataract surgery is extremely low. In a study of 19,557 elective cataract operations, there were only 3 deaths, 8 myocardial infarctions, and 13 clinically significant postoperative pulmonary complications in the entire study population.

Ophthalmologists perform cataract surgery as an outpatient procedure. Anesthesia consists of local anesthesia combined with conscious sedation. The choice of agents for conscious sedation is similar to that used for nonsurgical procedures, such as bronchoscopy or gastrointestinal endoscopy. Commonly used short-acting intravenous agents include methohexital and propofol. The physiologic stress and resulting cardiac risk of cataract surgery are similar to that of endoscopic procedures. The American College of Cardiology and American Heart Association preoperative cardiac risk assessment guideline acknowledges this low risk. The guideline classifies cataract surgery as low cardiac risk and groups this procedure with superficial procedures, endoscopic procedures, and breast surgery as having rates of cardiac complications that are generally <1%. From a standpoint of cardiac risk assessment, clinicians may approach the patient preparing for cataract surgery as they would the patient undergoing a nonsurgical procedure, such as gastrointestinal endoscopy.

A history and physical examination are the most important elements of the evaluation of patients before cataract surgery. The clinician seeks factors known to increase risk, such as a history of a bleeding diathesis, poor exercise capacity, or a recent change in anginal pattern. Cataract surgery poses no unique stresses or risks other than those associated with minor surgery and conscious sedation.

Cataract surgery is a procedure of the elderly. In this group of patients with higher than average medical comorbidities, it is understandable that physicians wish to stratify risk for these patients before surgery. Given the low baseline risk associated with cataract surgery, however, most potential preoperative laboratory tests fail to modify significantly risk assessment or outcomes. Historically, clinicians frequently have recommended more routine preoperative laboratory tests than are justified by the available literature. Cataract surgery is no exception. Several studies have shown great heterogeneity in the use of routine testing before cataract surgery and that ophthalmologists recommend more testing than do internists or anesthesiologists. More recently, several studies have provided compelling evidence that less is more with regard to laboratory testing before cataract surgery.

In the largest of these studies, researchers randomly assigned nearly 20,000 patients undergoing cataract surgery to routine testing, including ECG, CBC, serum electrolytes, BUN, creatinine, and glucose, or to no routine testing. No difference existed between the two groups in the rates of intraoperative complications, postoperative complications, cardiac complications, need for hospitalization, or death. The most common minor complications were hypertension and bradyarrhythmias; these occurred in 1.3% and 0.5% of patients. This study showed that preoperative testing did not reduce perioperative morbidity or mortality. In a subgroup analysis, this finding held true for high-risk patients with preexisting medical comorbidities and across all American Society of Anesthesiologists classes. The authors recommended that clinicians discard routine testing and reserve preoperative testing for patients who had an indication for testing independent of their need for cataract surgery. An example would be an ECG for a patient with a changed anginal pattern.

The present patient had stable exertional angina at a moderate workload by history and no factors that would increase his risk above average. He was taking no medications that require preoperative laboratory monitoring. Most clinicians would obtain an ECG given this patient's age and presumed coronary artery disease, although the literature would support an approach of clinical evaluation only without an ECG. The preoperative evaluation should include a history and physical examination. If no additional factors exist that would modify his risk, he could proceed to cataract surgery at average risk without the need for additional testing, other than possibly an ECG.

Clinical Pearls

1. Cataract surgery is safe and can be performed with an extremely low overall risk of perioperative mortality, hospitalization, and cardiac and pulmonary morbidities that is similar to that of endoscopic procedures.

2. The history and physical examination are the most important elements of the preoperative assessment before cataract surgery.

3. Routine preoperative laboratory testing does not identify a high-risk subset of patients, and it does not reduce the morbidity or mortality of cataract surgery.

4. Preoperative testing should be obtained only if an indication exists outside of the need for cataract surgery.

REFERENCES

1. Bellan L: Preoperative testing for cataract surgery. Can J Ophthalmol 29:111–114, 1994.
2. Bass EB, Steinberg EP, Luthra R, et al: Do ophthalmologists, anesthesiologists, and internists agree about preoperative testing in healthy patients undergoing cataract surgery? Arch Ophthalmol 113:1248–1256, 1995.
3. American College of Cardiology/American Heart Association task force on practice guidelines: Guidelines for perioperative cardiovascular evaluation for noncardiac surgery. Circulation 93:1278–1317, 1996.
4. Schein OD, Katz J, Bass EB, et al, for the Study of Medical Testing for Cataract Surgery: The value of routine preoperative medical testing before cataract surgery. N Engl J Med 342:168–175, 2000.

PATIENT 17

A 62-year-old woman with depression who is preparing for electroconvulsive therapy

A 62-year-old woman is hospitalized for depression that has become refractory to antidepressant medication. Her psychiatrist recommends electroconvulsive therapy (ECT) and requests a medical consultation to determine her risk of this procedure. She has a history of well-controlled hypertension and peptic ulcer disease. There is no known cardiac history. Exercise capacity is fair; she can walk 0.5 mile before stopping because of fatigue. She has occasional headaches. Her only medication is hydrochlorothiazide, 25 mg daily.

Physical Examination: Temperature 37°C, blood pressure 150/92, heart rate 72, respirations 12. Chest: clear. Cardiac: regular rhythm with no murmurs or rubs. Neurologic: alert and oriented, flat affect, cranial nerves II through XII normal, motor examination symmetric, gait and reflexes normal.

Laboratory Findings: ECG: normal. Head magnetic resonance imaging (MRI): normal (see Figure).

Question: How should the risk associated with ECT be assessed in this patient?

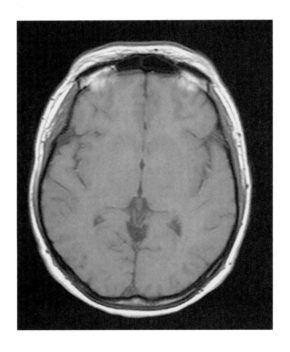

Answer: Assess risk in the same fashion as for surgery and anesthesia with the exception of special attention to risk of arrhythmia and to the possibility of increased intracranial pressure.

Discussion: Internists commonly perform medical consultations on patients admitted to inpatient psychiatric units; evaluation before ECT is one of the most common requests. Because ECT is particularly valuable for elderly depressed patients, issues often arise related to the impact of medical comorbidities on the risk of ECT. ECT is effective in 70% of patients with treatment-refractory depression. A course of treatment most commonly consists of 6 to 12 treatments over several weeks.

In ECT, electrical current is applied to one or both sides of the head after premedication with a short-acting intravenous anesthetic agent (commonly methohexital) and a neuromuscular blocker (commonly succinylcholine). Atropine often is administered to minimize the risk of bradycardia after the electrical impulse and to decrease secretions. The electrical current induces a generalized seizure. The use of neuromuscular blockers minimizes the risk of orthopedic injury; such injury was common in the early days of ECT before the use of paralyzing agents became standard. Mortality resulting from ECT is <4 per 100,000 treatments; this figure is similar to the mortality among American Society of Anesthesiologists class I patients undergoing ambulatory general surgery.

ECT causes parasympathetic stimulation followed by a period of adrenergic activity. The electrical discharge and resulting seizure lead to a vagal outpouring with bradycardia and relative hypotension for 60 seconds; a brief period of asystole may occur. A compensatory tachycardia and hypertension follow. Patients with underlying conduction disease may be at risk for either bradyarrhythmias or tachyarrhythmias. During the period of enhanced sympathetic tone, sinus tachycardia and hypertension may precipitate myocardial ischemia in susceptible patients; tachyarrhythmias may include atrial fibrillation, supraventricular tachycardia, and ventricular tachycardia.

β-Blockers blunt the effects of this sympathetic surge and should be used in patients with a history of tachyarrhythmias, coronary artery disease, and poorly controlled hypertension. Short-acting intravenous agents are given immediately before ECT; options include esmolol or labetalol. These agents also may be used to treat persistent post-ECT hypertension as part of the monitored anesthesia care. Both agents reduce the post-ECT increases in blood pressure and prevent the expected increase in heart rate. Although patients with preexisting cardiac disease have a higher incidence of complications than patients without cardiac disease, most cardiac complications of ECT are mild and transient and lead to no morbidity.

There are no absolute contraindications to ECT. The evaluation of patients before ECT is similar to the evaluation of patients who are preparing for general anesthesia and surgery and should include a history, physical examination, and ECG. Cardiac risk indices, such as the Goldman or revised cardiac risk index, stratify the risk of cardiac complications of ECT. Using these indices, relative contraindications to ECT include myocardial infarction within the past 6 months, uncompensated congestive heart failure, and significant aortic stenosis.

Another relative contraindication to ECT is increased intracranial pressure. In a patient with new-onset progressive depression, in whom an occult mass lesion in the brain is possible, one should obtain a head MRI study before ECT. A screening neurologic examination should be part of every pre-ECT evaluation; unexplained abnormalities also should prompt head MRI. It is not necessary to obtain neuroimaging routinely in all patients before ECT. Patients with primary headaches (migraine, tension-type headache) whose headache pattern does not suggest the possibility of a new pathologic cause of headache may undergo ECT safely. In approximately 20% of patients, preexisting headaches may worsen or new headaches may develop after ECT. A recent stroke is also a relative contraindication to ECT.

In the present patient, there was no history of cardiac disease that would increase her risk. Her hypertension was suboptimally controlled, and she would benefit from the use of a short-acting intravenous β-blocker to blunt the hypertensive response to ECT. The clinician should inquire about the nature of her headaches. If they were new, progressive, or otherwise worrisome for intracranial pathology, a head MRI study should be obtained to exclude a mass lesion before proceeding to ECT.

Clinical Pearls

1. ECT is a safe procedure for patients with preexisting cardiac disease.

2. Medical consultation for patients before ECT is similar to the estimation of risk before general anesthesia and surgery. Recent myocardial infarction, uncompensated congestive heart failure, and aortic stenosis are relative contraindications to ECT.

3. Parasympathetic and sympathetic surges occur after ECT and lead to a risk of bradyarrhythmias and subsequent tachyarrhythmias, hypertension, and myocardial ischemia.

4. Short-acting intravenous β-blockers should be used immediately before ECT in patients with a history of coronary artery disease, poorly controlled hypertension, and tachyarrhythmias. Pretreatment with atropine minimizes the risk of bradycardia immediately after ECT in patients treated with β-blockers.

5. Recent stroke and increased intracranial pressure are relative contraindications to ECT.

REFERENCES

1. Crowe RR: Electroconvulsive therapy—current perspective. N Engl J Med 311:163–167, 1984.
2. Gaines GY, Rees DI: Anesthetic considerations for electroconvulsive therapy. South Med J 85:469–482, 1992.
3. Zielinski RJ, Roose SP, Devanand DP, et al: Cardiovascular complications of ECT in depressed patients with cardiac disease. Am J Pyschiatry 150:904–909, 1993.
4. Weiner SJ, Ward TN, Ravaris CL: Headache and electroconvulsive therapy. Headache 34:155–159, 1994.
5. de Silva RA, Bachman WR: Cardiac consultation in patients with neuropsychiatric problems. Cardiol Clin 13:225–239, 1995.
6. Kelly KG, Zisselman M: Update on electroconvulsive therapy (ECT) in older adults. J Am Geriatr Soc 45:560–566, 2000.

PATIENT 18

**A 42-year-old woman presenting for preoperative testing
before arthroscopic repair of a meniscal tear**

A 42-year-old woman has sustained an injury to her right knee while running and has developed pain and clicking. Magnetic resonance imaging confirms a meniscal tear, and she is scheduled for elective arthroscopic repair. Past medical history is negative. Before her injury, she could run for 5 miles with no dyspnea or other exercise intolerance. She takes no regular medications.

Physical Examination: Blood pressure 130/78, heart rate 62, respirations 12. HEENT: normal. Chest: clear. Cardiac: regular rate and rhythm, no murmurs, gallops, or rubs.

Laboratory Findings: Deferred.

Question: What routine laboratory tests should be obtained in this healthy woman preparing for surgery?

Answer: None. The history and physical examination are the primary tools to stratify perioperative risk in healthy patients.

Discussion: Perioperative morbidity and mortality in healthy patients is low. Mortality for otherwise healthy patients undergoing surgery (American Society of Anesthesiologists class I) has varied from 0% to 0.07% in the literature. Given the low morbidity, attempts at risk stratification through the use of routine preoperative laboratory testing generally add little information.

Tradition has led to recommendations for routine testing panels. Most of these test results were ignored before surgery, and abnormal test results were more likely to be false-positives than true-positives. This situation is due to the low prevalence of the screened conditions in the healthy asymptomatic population. More recently, an evidence-based approach has allowed a more thoughtful approach to the selective use of preoperative testing.

For a preoperative screening test to be useful in unselected patients, it must screen for a condition that is common and contributes to perioperative morbidity if unrecognized and untreated. An inexpensive test must be available with high sensitivity and low morbidity to the patient. Evidence must exist that identification and treatment of the condition in the asymptomatic patient before surgery reduces the risk of perioperative morbidity. There should be a long interval between the development of a positive screening test result and the development of clinically apparent disease. Relatively few tests meet these strict criteria. Standards of practice are based to some extent on expert opinion rather than unequivocal evidence.

Although physician concern about medicolegal liability may drive some routine laboratory screening, even this rationale seems to be unwarranted. Such routine testing panels may deviate from local standards of care, and an unordered test may pose less risk than an abnormal test result that is ignored.

Many tests that commonly were performed in the past have a low yield in the identification of clinically inapparent disease that benefits from preoperative recognition and treatment. In a now classic study by Kaplan et al in 1985, only 0.22% of routine preoperative laboratory tests among 2000 patients revealed abnormalities that might have influenced perioperative management, and none of these abnormalities resulted in change in treatment or influenced outcomes. In other words, not a single patient benefited from routine preoperative laboratory testing. Several other authors have reported similar results. When laboratory tests have been performed recently, normal test results obtained within 4 months before surgery may be used safely as preoperative tests unless there has been a change in the patient's condition in the interval.

Routine **chest radiographs** infrequently lead to improved patient outcomes. In a meta-analysis of 21 studies of preoperative chest radiographs that included a total of 14,390 patients, there were only 140 unexpected abnormalities. Only 14 radiographs (0.1% of total) were unexpected, were abnormal, and influenced management. In another report, authors validated a model that predicted a higher likelihood of abnormal screening preoperative chest radiographs. Based on this model, they recommended chest radiographs for patients with three or more risk factors among bronchopulmonary factors, cardiovascular factors, and an abnormal cardiopulmonary physical examination. Based on these and other reports, clinicians should obtain a preoperative chest radiograph in patients whose history or physical examination suggests cardiac or pulmonary disease. Data are insufficient for a firm recommendation on older individuals without such risk factors; most experts recommend a chest radiograph in healthy patients >60 years old.

The purpose of a routine **ECG** is to identify a patient at higher than average risk for postoperative cardiac complications. Q waves not known to have been present for at least 6 months, rhythm other than sinus, premature atrial contractions, and frequent premature ventricular contractions are such findings. Reports have cast doubt on the value of routine preoperative ECGs and have found them to have limited ability to stratify risk of adverse cardiac outcomes. Most experts still adhere to the indications first suggested by Goldberger and O'Konski: (1) history or physical findings suggesting heart disease, (2) men >45 years old and women >55 years old; (3) systemic disease that increases the likelihood of cardiovascular disease (e.g., diabetes); (4) use of medications that increase the likelihood of electrolyte abnormalities; and (5) use of medications with potential cardiac toxicity.

Summary recommendations for individual laboratory tests are given in the Table. These recommendations apply to healthy patients. Additional indications exist for patients with medical conditions known to increase the likelihood of an abnormal result.

The present patient was in excellent overall health. She did not need a routine ECG or chest radiograph. She would need a pregnancy test if pregnancy could not be excluded after taking a history. No additional laboratory testing would be necessary.

Suggested Indications for Routine Preoperative Laboratory Tests in Healthy Patients Who Take No Medications and Have No Known Medical Conditions

Test	Indication
Hct	Any surgery in which blood loss is likely
WBC count	No indication
Urinalysis	No indication
Serum glucose	No indication
Bleeding tests	Only if history suggests a bleeding tendency
Serum creatinine	All patients >50 years old and any patient in whom perioperative hypotension is likely
Electrolytes	No indication
Liver function tests	No indication
Pregnancy testing	All women in whom pregnancy cannot be excluded by history
Chest radiograph	Cardiac or pulmonary disease suspected after history and physical examination
	All patients >60 years old undergoing major surgery
ECG	Cardiac disease suspected after history and physical examination
	All men >45 years old
	All women >55 years old

Adapted from Smetana GW: Preoperative assessment of the healthy patient. In Braunwald E, Fauci AS, Isselbacher KJ, et al (eds): Harrison's Principles of Internal Medicine, online edition. New York, McGraw-Hill, 2000; with permission.

Clinical Pearls

1. Morbidity and mortality for healthy patients undergoing surgery are low.
2. Results of routine preoperative laboratory testing rarely influence management, and many abnormal results are false-positive results.
3. Physicians should perform preoperative laboratory testing selectively based on patient factors and the type of proposed surgery.

REFERENCES

1. Kaplan EB, Sheiner LB, Boeckmann AJ, et al: The usefulness of preoperative laboratory screening. JAMA 253:3576–3581, 1985.
2. Goldberger AL, O'Konski M: Utility of the routine electrocardiogram before surgery and on general hospital admission. Ann Intern Med 105:552–557, 1986.
3. Macpherson DS, Snow R, Lofgen RP: Preoperative screening: Value of previous tests. Ann Intern Med 113:969–973, 1990.
4. Archer C, Levy AR, McGregor M: Value of routine preoperative chest x-rays: A meta-analysis. Can J Anaesth 40:1022–1027, 1993.
5. Bouillot JL, Fingerhut A, Paquet JC, et al: Are routine preoperative chest radiographs useful in general surgery? Eur J Surg 162:597–604, 1996.
6. Smetana GW: Preoperative assessment of the healthy patient. In Braunwald E, Fauci AS, Isselbacher KJ, et al (eds): Harrison's Online. New York, McGraw-Hill, 2000. Available at http://harrisonsonline.com.

PATIENT 19

A 77-year-old man presenting for preoperative evaluation
before abdominal aortic aneurysm repair

A 77-year-old man is found to have a pulsatile abdominal mass on routine physical examination that subsequently is confirmed to be a 6-cm abdominal aortic aneurysm. He has stable bilateral claudication at one block level ground but no history of chest pain, exertional dyspnea, or known cardiac disease. Past medical history also includes hypertension and insulin-dependent diabetes. Medications are hydrochlorothiazide, amlodipine, NPH insulin, and regular insulin.

Physical Examination: Temperature 98.6°F, blood pressure 150/86, heart rate 72, respirations 12. Chest: clear. Cardiac: Regular rhythm, normal S_1 and S_2; S_4 present. No S_3, murmur, rub, or jugular venous distention. Abdomen: palpable aortic pulsation, which is widened in the upper abdomen. Extremities: no edema.

Laboratory Findings: ECG: normal sinus rhythm at 70, left ventricular hypertrophy but otherwise normal. Abdominal ultrasound: 6-cm infrarenal abdominal aortic aneurysm.

Question: How does the clinician estimate the risk of perioperative cardiac complications in this patient preparing for major vascular surgery?

Answer: Use a combination of clinical risk factors and pharmacologic stress testing to estimate cardiac risk.

Discussion: Patients undergoing vascular surgery have a high risk for perioperative cardiac complications. Peripheral vascular disease is a marker for generalized atherosclerosis and predicts a higher than average likelihood of coronary artery disease (CAD), even when no symptoms of CAD are apparent. In a classic angiographic study of 1000 patients with peripheral vascular disease before vascular reconstructive surgery, 31% of patients had severe CAD, whereas only 8% had completely normal coronary arteries. As a result of the high prevalence of CAD in this group of patients, clinical risk indices, which were derived from general surgical populations, fail to identify a low-risk group. A low score on the Goldman, Detsky, or revised cardiac risk index does not result in a low risk of perioperative cardiac complications. In contrast, a high score on one of these cardiac risk indices does predict a high risk of complications. An additional factor that limits the use of clinical criteria to estimate risk is the frequent occurrence of claudication in these patients. Claudication may limit activity in a patient who otherwise would display symptoms of myocardial ischemia, such as angina, if he or she were able to walk further.

Given the failure of risk indices to identify a low-risk population, investigators have evaluated several noninvasive testing strategies to predict risk more accurately. Early attempts to use preoperative silent ischemia on ambulatory electrographic monitoring (Holter monitoring) proved to be unsuccessful, and this test no longer is recommended. The two tests with the most evidence of predictive value are dipyridamole thallium testing and dobutamine stress echocardiography (DSE). Dipyridamole thallium testing involves the injection of intravenous thallium. At high doses, dipyridamole is a coronary vasodilator. This vasodilation leads to a *coronary steal* phenomenon. Healthy coronary arteries vasodilate, but there can be no vasodilation at points of fixed coronary stenoses. Blood preferentially flows to normal vascular beds. Thallium testing shows relative reduction in blood flow past fixed coronary lesions. A positive test also may result in chest pain or ECG changes of ischemia, but these generally are not considered in interpreting the results.

DSE involves the incremental infusion of dobutamine intravenously. A positive test is a new or worsened wall motion abnormality. Both tests have similar test characteristics. The negative predictive values are high and are generally in the 95% to 100% range in different studies. A negative result predicts a low risk of complications. The positive predictive values are low, however, at 10% to 20%. If one chose to proceed to invasive cardiac evaluation for all patients with a positive test result, many would be subjected to additional risk, whereas only a few patients would have had an event in the first place.

The solution to this dilemma is the incorporation of clinical risk factors or predictors into an algorithm for the use of pharmacologic stress testing. The most widely cited strategy is that of Eagle et al. They evaluated clinical variables including Q waves on ECG, age >70 years, history of angina, history of ventricular ectopic activity requiring treatment, and diabetes requiring treatment. Among 200 study patients undergoing vascular surgery, patients with no clinical variables had a low risk of events (3.1%). The investigators concluded that these patients needed no additional testing. Patients with three or more of the five clinical risk factors had a high risk (50%). These patients can be presumed to be at high risk without the need for additional testing. The patients with one or two clinical variables had an intermediate risk and benefited most from additional testing. Patients with a negative dipyridamole thallium study had the same risk as the patients with no clinical variables, whereas patients with a positive study had a high risk (29.6%) that approached the risk of the patients with three or more clinical variables. The use of such a scheme, which incorporates clinical predictors, improves the predictive value of pharmacologic stress testing.

A group evaluating the benefit of perioperative β-blockers in vascular surgery patients used the revised cardiac risk index of Lee et al to aid in the selection of candidates for noninvasive testing with DSE. They found that when perioperative β-blockers were used to reduce cardiac risk, only patients with three or more of six clinical risk factors benefited from DSE testing. These factors included age ≥70 years, current angina, prior myocardial infarction, congestive heart failure, prior cerebrovascular event, diabetes, and renal failure.

The American College of Physicians position statement on preoperative cardiac risk assessment has endorsed this approach as the recommended strategy for risk stratification before vascular surgery. The American College of Cardiology guideline also incorporates clinical predictors to determine which patients would benefit from additional testing, although it cites different factors than the original Eagle criteria.

The present patient was >70 years old and had diabetes requiring treatment. According to the Eagle criteria, he had two of five clinical variables and should have had a pharmacologic stress test to stratify the risk of cardiac complications. Either a DSE or dipyridamole thallium test can be done, depending on the skill of the test operators at an individual institution.

Clinical Pearls

1. Patients undergoing major vascular surgery have a high incidence of perioperative cardiac complications as a result of a high likelihood of coexisting CAD.

2. A low score on a cardiac risk index does not predict a low risk of cardiac events for patients undergoing major vascular surgery.

3. Pharmacologic stress testing using either dipyridamole thallium or DSE stratifies risk of cardiac complications.

4. Such testing should be reserved for patients with an intermediate number of clinical risk factors for complications.

REFERENCES

1. Hertzer NR, Beven EG, Young JR, et al: Coronary artery disease in peripheral vascular patients: A classification of 1000 coronary angiograms and results of surgical management. Ann Surg 199:223–233, 1984.
2. Eagle KA, Coley CM, Newell JB, et al: Combining clinical and thallium data optimizes preoperative assessment of cardiac risk before major vascular surgery. Ann Intern Med 110:859–866, 1989.
3. American College of Cardiology/American Heart Association task force on practice guidelines: Guidelines for perioperative cardiovascular evaluation for noncardiac surgery. Circulation 93:1278–1317, 1996.
4. American College of Physicians: Guidelines for assessing and managing the perioperative cardiac risk from coronary artery disease associated with major noncardiac surgery. Ann Intern Med 127:309–312, 1997.
5. Boersma E, Poldermans D, Bax JJ, et al: Predictors of cardiac events after major vascular surgery. JAMA 285:1865–1873, 2001.

PATIENT 20

A 64-year-old woman with a recent myocardial infarction and a new diagnosis of colon cancer

A 64-year-old woman sustained a non–Q wave myocardial infarction (MI) 6 weeks ago. At that time, she underwent emergent direct angioplasty of an occluded left anterior descending artery. There was subcritical disease in the other coronary arteries. Her peak creatine kinase value was 434 IU/L. A post-MI ECG showed no Q waves. On medical therapy, she has been asymptomatic since. She is able to walk 1 mile without chest pain or shortness of breath. Last week, in evaluation of occult blood in the stool and abdominal pain, she was found to have a malignancy in the descending colon. Her surgeon wishes to resect this tumor and requests a consultation to determine the timing of surgery. Past medical history includes hypertension and elevated cholesterol. Medications are atenolol, atorvastatin, aspirin, and lisinopril.

Physical Examination: Blood pressure 134/82, heart rate 52. Chest: clear. Cardiac: regular rhythm, normal S_1S_2 with an S_4. No S_3, murmur, rub, or jugular venous distention. Abdomen: no masses, tenderness, or hepatosplenomegaly.

Laboratory Findings: CBC: Hct 34%, WBC 5400/μL. Blood chemistries normal. ECG: see Figure (next page).

Questions: What is the risk of proceeding to noncardiac surgery 6 weeks after a MI? How might this risk be minimized?

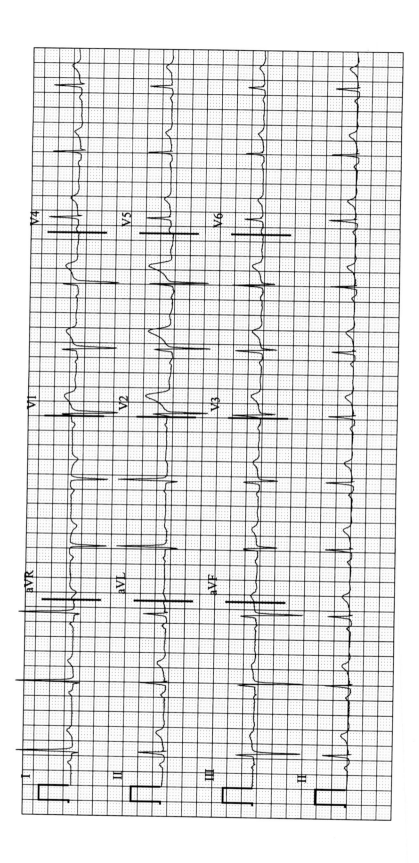

Answers: Cardiac risk is highest in the first 6 months after MI. Risk stratification and perioperative β-blockers modify risk.

Discussion: One of the earliest observations in the study of perioperative cardiac risk was that patients who had sustained a MI within the previous 6 months had a high risk of reinfarction in the perioperative period. This finding dates to the early 1970s in a classic paper from the Mayo Clinic. In that study, overall perioperative infarction rate was 0.13%. Among patients with a recent MI, reinfarction rates were 37% for patients with a MI within the past 3 months, 16% for patients with a MI 3 to 6 months previously, and 5% for patients with a MI >6 months previously. The mortality among patients who suffered a reinfarction was high (54%). Other groups since have shown similar results: The risk of reinfarction is highest in the first 6 months after MI. Absolute risks have been lower, however, in studies performed in the modern era.

In the landmark original cardiac risk index of Goldman et al, a MI within the past 6 months was one of the two strongest predictors of perioperative MI (the other being S_3 or jugular venous distention). Based on these and other observations, most clinicians have recommended deferring all but emergent surgery for patients who have had a MI within the previous 6 months. No similar studies exist of the risk of reinfarction in the modern era of thrombolysis and direct angioplasty. Mortality and short-term prognosis are improved by urgent revascularization for acute MI. It is likely that these patients, with a lower incidence of inducible ischemia in the post-MI period than patients with conservatively managed MIs, also have a lower risk in the event of noncardiac surgery. No authors have studied, however, the risk of perioperative infarction in the first 6 months after a MI that has been aborted by thrombolysis or direct angioplasty.

In practice, semiurgent surgical indications often arise. These surgeries are not emergent but are not entirely elective. Commonly, these are surgeries to resect potentially curable cancers, for which a delay of 6 months potentially could decrease the likelihood of cure. In these cases, such as the present patient, risk stratification can identify patients who may proceed to noncardiac surgery with an acceptable risk. In a patient with a recent MI who has not already been studied, a functional assessment of residual ischemia is helpful. Patients who are able to exercise to a good workload (rate pressure product of 20,000 or at least 85% of age-predicted maximal heart rate) on an exercise tolerance test have a favorable prognosis after MI. Because the stress of surgery and anesthesia generally are no greater than this degree of effort, it is likely that these patients also can undergo noncardiac surgery with an acceptable risk. Patients with ischemia at a lower workload on exercise testing are at higher risk. For these patients, surgery should be delayed if possible, unless this degree of risk is acceptable to the patient and surgeon when balanced with the potential benefit of surgery. No data prove that revascularization of such patients reduces the risk of subsequent perioperative cardiac events.

The risk for these patients is still greater than for patients without known cardiac disease. In the revised cardiac risk index of Lee et al, any symptomatic coronary artery disease is a risk factor; this risk is not limited to patients with a recent MI. It is unlikely, however, that further delay of surgery for the patient with a recent aborted MI and subsequent absence of inducible ischemia would reduce risk to an additional degree.

If after risk stratification one elects to proceed to noncardiac surgery within the first 6 months after MI, the most important strategy to reduce risk is the use of perioperative β-blockers. Validated protocols include the use of perioperative atenolol and the use of oral bisoprolol beginning 1 week before surgery and continued until 1 month after surgery. It is likely that any β-blocker would reduce risk as long as intravenous forms also are used in the immediate perioperative period as necessary to maintain the heart rate <80 beats/min.

In the present patient, the history suggested a favorable post-MI prognosis given the good exercise capacity. If the patient and surgeon wished to proceed before 6 months had elapsed since her MI, an exercise tolerance test should be recommended to stratify her risk further. If the patient exercised to a good workload with no ischemia, she could proceed to surgery with the use of a perioperative β-blocker protocol. Although incomplete evidence exists for this strategy in the modern era of treatment of acute MI, it is a reasonable approach.

Clinical Pearls

1. MI within the past 6 months is a major risk factor for perioperative cardiac complications.

2. It is unknown whether the same risk exists in the modern era of thrombolysis and direct angioplasty for the treatment of MI, but the risk is probably less.

3. If a patient needs semiurgent surgery during this 6-month period, risk should be stratified by a functional test, such as an exercise tolerance test. Patients with a favorable-prognosis stress test probably also have a lower risk of perioperative cardiac complications for subsequent noncardiac surgery.

4. Perioperative β-blockers should be used in any patient who needs surgery in the post-MI period.

REFERENCES

1. Tarhan S, Moffitt EA, Taylor WF, Giuliani ER: Myocardial infarction after general anesthesia. JAMA 220:1451–1454, 1972.
2. Goldman L, Caldera DL, Nussbaum SR, et al: Multifactorial index of cardiac risk in noncardiac surgical procedures. N Engl J Med 297:845–850, 1977.
3. Steen PA, Tinker JH, Tarhan S: Myocardial reinfarction after anesthesia and surgery. JAMA 239:2566–2570, 1978.
4. Rao TK, Jacobs KH, El-Etr AA: Reinfarction following anesthesia in patients with myocardial infarction. Anesthesiology 59:499–505, 1983.
5. Lee TH, Marcantonio ER, Mangione CM, et al: Derivation and prospective validation of a simple index for prediction of cardiac risk of major noncardiac surgery. Circulation 100:1043–1049, 1999.

PATIENT 21

An 81-year-old woman with chest pain and ECG changes after cholecystectomy

An 81-year-old woman was admitted to the hospital 2 days ago for fever and right upper quadrant pain and yesterday underwent open cholecystectomy for acute cholecystitis. A laparoscopic approach was not recommended because of prior abdominal surgery and concern for adhesions. She received no specific pharmacologic treatment to reduce perioperative cardiac risk. Her perioperative course has been uncomplicated until 1 day postsurgery when she develops chest pain and shortness of breath. Past medical history includes hypertension, a previous hysterectomy for uterine fibroids, and gastro-esophageal reflux disease. Medications are hydrochlorothiazide and ranitidine.

Physical Examination: Temperature 99.2°F, blood pressure 180/86, heart rate 76, respirations 20. Chest: clear. Cardiac: tachycardic, regular rhythm, S_1S_2 with an S_4. No S_3 or murmur. Jugular venous pressure normal.

Laboratory Findings: CBC: Hct 32%, WBC 11,300/μL. Creatine kinase 1224 IU/L. ECG (see Figure): ST depressions in V1-V3, 1 mm. ST elevation in II, III, and aVF.

Questions: What is the cause of the patient's postoperative symptoms? How is the condition diagnosed, and what is the treatment?

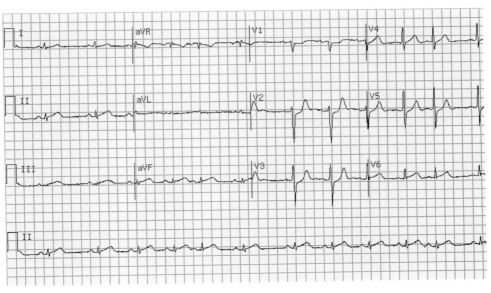

Courtesy of ECG Wave-Maven, Boston, MA

Answer: Postoperative myocardial infarction (MI). When postoperative MI is suspected, the diagnosis and treatment are the same as for nonoperative infarctions.

Discussion: Cardiac complications are the source of the greatest morbidity of surgery and anesthesia. The most important complications that clinicians seek to prevent are postoperative MI, congestive heart failure, arrhythmia, and cardiac death. The mortality of postoperative MI is much higher than that of MI occurring in the nonoperative setting. Postoperative MIs often present atypically. In contrast to nonoperative MIs, presenting features more commonly include dyspnea, arrhythmia, and hypotension. Many postoperative MIs are asymptomatic. Previous studies had identified postoperative days 3 through 5 as being a particularly high-risk period; this was thought to be due to increasing ambulation, fluid mobilization, and reduction of pain medication. A more recent study has concluded otherwise.

Authors prospectively studied 323 patients with known coronary artery disease undergoing noncardiac surgery with serial creatine kinase and troponin measurements, daily ECGs, and clinical assessment. Eighteen patients had perioperative MIs. Only eight patients had chest pain, whereas nine patients had shortness of breath or heart failure. Four patients presented only with hypotension, two presented with atrial fibrillation, and two were asymptomatic. The period of peak risk for perioperative MI, in contrast to earlier reports, was on the day of surgery, and risk extended until postoperative day 2. Only one MI occurred after postoperative day 2.

In a similar prospective study of patients undergoing noncardiac surgery, investigators performed routine surveillance for postoperative MIs by obtaining daily ECGs and creatine kinase measurement. These study patients had varied risk for cardiac events, and not all patients had known coronary artery disease. The overall incidence of postoperative MI was 1.7%; that among patients with known coronary artery disease was 4.1%. Two thirds (10 of 15) of the postoperative MIs occurred on or before the third postoperative day. Chest pain was the presenting symptom in only 2 of the 15 patients who sustained a postoperative MI, and 3 patients were asymptomatic.

Clinicians should have a high index of suspicion for postoperative MI and consider this diagnosis in the presence of postoperative chest pain, dyspnea, hypotension, or arrhythmia. Because perioperative β-blockers substantially reduce the risk of postoperative MI for patients with known coronary artery disease or at least two risk factors for coronary artery disease, the clinician should be especially diligent in considering the possibility of postoperative MI when asked to evaluate a patient with any of these features who did not appropriately receive perioperative β-blockers.

The treatment of postoperative MI is the same as for nonoperative MI. An exception is the potential for contraindication to thrombolysis depending on the nature of the surgical procedure and the ability to control bleeding complications. For most procedures other than trivial superficial procedures, thrombolysis should be avoided, and direct angiography and angioplasty is the preferred approach for urgent revascularization.

The present patient presented more typically with chest pain on the first postoperative day. Her ECG showed changes consistent with ischemia. If nitrates, β-blockers, and aspirin do not promptly relieve her pain and ECG changes, she should be suspected of having a perioperative MI. Treatment would include an urgent angiogram and possible direct angioplasty.

Clinical Pearls

1. Presenting features of postoperative myocardial infarction are often atypical and include dyspnea, hypotension, or arrhythmia.

2. Postoperative MIs occur most frequently on the day of surgery and the first two postoperative days.

3. The treatment of postoperative MI is generally the same as that for infarctions in the nonoperative setting.

4. An important difference in the treatment of postoperative MI is the relative *contraindication of thrombolysis* due to the risk of bleeding at the surgical site.

REFERENCES

1. Ashton CM, Petersen NJ, Wray NP, et al: The incidence of perioperative myocardial infarction in men undergoing noncardiac surgery. Ann Intern Med 118:504–510, 1993.
2. Badner NH, Knill RL, Brown JE, et al: Myocardial infarction after noncardiac surgery. Anesthesiology 88:572–578, 1998.

PATIENT 22

A 72-year-old man preparing for gastrectomy

A 72-year-old man is seen for routine preoperative evaluation before gastrectomy for a gastric adenocarcinoma and for estimation of cardiac risk. He is able to walk only two blocks before stopping because of fatigue and dyspnea. He reports no history of chest pain or known cardiac disease. Past medical history includes hypertension and chronic renal insufficiency resulting from diabetic nephropathy. Medications are lisinopril, ranitidine, and glyburide.

Physical Examination: Temperature 98.4°F, blood pressure 140/88, heart rate 76, respirations 14. General appearance: a chronically ill–appearing man in no respiratory distress at rest. Chest: clear. Cardiac: S_1S_2 with an S_4; no S_3 or murmur. Abdomen: soft, nontender, no masses or hepatosplenomegaly.

Laboratory Findings: CBC: Hct 39%, WBC 5700/μL. Electrolytes: sodium 141, potassium 5.0, chloride 112, bicarbonate 22, BUN 60, creatinine 3.2. Chest radiograph: normal. ECG: sinus rhythm at 72; normal intervals, axis, and morphology.

Question: How can the risk of postoperative cardiac complications in this patient be estimated?

Answer: Cardiac risk can be estimated through the use of established cardiac risk indices and integrative guidelines.

Discussion: An assessment of cardiac risk should be part of every medical consultation before surgery. Cardiac and pulmonary complications are the most important sources of perioperative morbidity. The major cardiac complications are postoperative myocardial infarction, arrhythmia, congestive heart failure, and cardiac death.

The science of preoperative cardiac risk stratification began with the work of Goldman et al with the first published cardiac risk index in 1977 (see Table below). In a study of 1001 patients undergoing noncardiac surgery, risk factors were tabulated; each was assigned a number of points based on its strength as a predictor in a multivariate analysis. An index was developed that stratified risk based on total number of points. Major predictors included congestive heart failure (S_3

Goldman Cardiac Risk Index

Variable	Points
History	
Age > 70 years old	5
MI in previous 6 mo	10
Physical examination	
S_3 gallop or jugular venous distention	11
Important valvular aortic stenosis	3
ECG	
Rhythm other than sinus or premature atrial contractions on last preoperative ECG	7
PVCs >5/min documented at any time before operation	7
General medical status	
PO_2 < 60 or PCO_2 > 50 mmHg, $K+$ < 3 or HCO_3 < 20, BUN > 50 or creatinine > 3, signs of chronic liver disease or patient bedridden from noncardiac causes	3
Operation	
Intraperitoneal, intrathoracic, or aortic	3
Emergency	4
Total possible points	53
Class I	0–5
Class II	6–12
Class III	13–25
Class IV	>25

PVC = premature ventricular contraction

Adapted from Goldman L, Cadera, DL, Nussbaum SR, et al: Multifactorial index of cardiac risk in noncardiac surgical procedures. N Engl J. Med 297:845–850,1977.

and jugular venous distention in particular) and myocardial infarction within the past 6 months. Intermediate predictors were age >70 years and atrial or ventricular arrhythmia. Minor factors included aortic stenosis; metabolic abnormalities; emergency surgery; and chest, abdominal, or aortic procedures. Other studies have validated the predictive value of this index. Detsky et al published a revised cardiac risk index, based on Goldman's index, which is the starting point for the American College of Physicians guideline.

Lee et al reported the findings of a revised cardiac risk index that outperformed the original Goldman index (see Table below). This index is simpler to use; each of six factors is assigned one point. New factors in this index include the recognition of the importance of diabetes requiring treatment and a history of symptomatic cerebrovascular disease. In addition, any clinical evidence of ischemic heart disease was a risk factor; risk was not limited to patients with recent myocardial infarction. This index was published after the completion of the principal consensus guidelines and so is not included in the guidelines. It is an easier index to use, however, than the original Goldman index and is a better risk predictor.

Two national organizations have reviewed the cardiac risk assessment literature and have published guidelines. Of the two, the American College of Physicians guideline is more clinically based and easier for clinicians to follow. This

Revised Cardiac Risk Index

Risk Factors
1. High-risk surgery
2. Ischemic heart disease
3. History of congestive heart failure
4. History of cerebrovascular disease
5. Insulin therapy for diabetes
6. Serum creatinine >2.0 mg/dL

Class	No. Points	Cardiac Complications (%) in Validation Cohort
I	0	0.4
II	1	0.9
III	2	6.6
IV	>2	11.0

Adapted from Lee TH, Marcantonio ER, Mangione CM, et al: Derivation and prospective validation of a simple index for prediction of cardiac risk of major noncardiac surgery. Circulation 100:1043–1049, 1999.

guideline recommends the use of the modified Detsky index as a starting point. Low-risk patients undergoing vascular surgery are stratified further by the use of the Eagle criteria; the guidelines recommend pharmacologic stress testing for intermediate-risk patients undergoing vascular surgery. High-risk patients by this algorithm should receive perioperative β-blockers, and risk should be reduced as appropriate to the nature of the high factor. Low-risk patients undergoing nonvascular surgery need no further testing.

The American College of Cardiology and American Heart Association guideline is more angiographically based in its initial triage. Initial steps inquire about recent revascularization and coronary evaluation. Subsequent branch points in the algorithm are based on, in order, clinical risk predictors, functional capacity, and surgery-specific risks. This guideline advances the field by the recognition of the importance of functional capacity as a predictor and the more refined estimate of surgery-specific risks than present in the other indices and guidelines. The guideline itself is complicated, however, with eight separate steps, and not easily committed to memory. A study has confirmed the predictive value of functional capacity. Patients who, by their own self-report, were unable to walk at least four blocks on level ground or climb two flights of stairs without symptoms had higher rates of overall and cardiac complications of surgery.

In the era of routine use of perioperative β-blockers for high-risk patients, certain elements of the risk stratification algorithms may prove to be less useful, other than for the goal of identifying very high risk patients for whom one may consider canceling surgery or revascularization based on considerations other than the impending noncardiac surgery. Clinicians may choose to design a risk stratification strategy that includes several of the published guidelines and indices. A reasonable strategy is to begin with the revised cardiac risk index, then to apply the Eagle criteria or the American College of Physicians guidelines to patients undergoing vascular surgery who are at low risk by the revised index.

The present patient was undergoing high-risk surgery (abdominal) and had a serum creatinine >2.0 mg/dL for a total of two out of six points in the revised cardiac risk index. Although the patient did have diabetes, he was not taking insulin, so this would not confer an additional point. He would be in the revised cardiac risk index class III and would be at moderately high risk with an estimated risk of cardiac complications of 6.6%. Because he was undergoing nonvascular surgery, one would not need to stratify risk further using the Eagle criteria.

Clinical Pearls

1. The clinician should use a cardiac risk index for the estimation of risk of postoperative cardiac complications.

2. The revised cardiac risk index of Lee et al offers simplicity and superior predictive value to previously published indices.

3. The clinician should apply the American College of Physicians guideline to patients at intermediate and high risk by the revised cardiac risk index.

4. The Eagle criteria can be used to stratify further low-risk patients undergoing vascular surgery.

REFERENCES

1. Goldman L, Caldera DL, Nussbaum SR, et al: Multifactorial index of cardiac risk in noncardiac surgical procedures. N Engl J Med 297:845–850, 1977.
2. Detsky AS, Abrams HB, Forbath N, et al: Cardiac assessment for patients undergoing noncardiac surgery: A multifactorial clinical risk index. Arch Intern Med 146:2131–2134, 1986.
3. American College of Cardiology/American Heart Association task force on practice guidelines: Guidelines for perioperative cardiovascular evaluation for noncardiac surgery. Circulation 93:1278–1317, 1996.
4. American College of Physicians: Guidelines for assessing and managing the perioperative cardiac risk from coronary artery disease associated with major noncardiac surgery. Ann Intern Med 127:309–312, 1997.
5. Lee TH, Marcantonio ER, Mangione CM, et al: Derivation and prospective validation of a simple index for prediction of cardiac risk of major noncardiac surgery. Circulation 100:1043–1049, 1999.
6. Reilly DF, McNeely MJ, Doerner D, et al: Self-reported exercise tolerance and the risk of serious perioperative complications. Arch Intern Med 159:2185–2192, 1999.

PATIENT 23

A 67-year-old woman with steroid-requiring polymyalgia rheumatica preparing for total knee replacement

A 67-year-old woman is seen in the preoperative medical consultation clinic 1 week before planned right total knee replacement for severe osteoarthritis. She is unable to walk >50 feet without knee pain. Past medical history includes polymyalgia rheumatica, which first was diagnosed 6 months ago. She was treated with prednisone, 10 mg daily, at that time. Her dose has been slowly tapered, although it was increased to 15 mg daily 3 weeks ago because of increased shoulder stiffness. She is otherwise in good health without other chronic medical conditions. Her only medications at present are prednisone, 15 mg daily, and ibuprofen, 600 mg three times daily as needed.

Physical Examination: Blood pressure 132/84, heart rate 72, respirations 14. General appearance: A well-appearing woman in no acute distress. Chest: clear. Cardiac: regular rate and rhythm, normal S_1S_2 without murmurs, rubs, or gallops. Extremities: bony deformity of both knees, right greater than left, with pain on range of motion and crepitus but no effusion or instability.

Laboratory Findings: CBC normal, electrolytes normal. ECG: normal.

Questions: Is this patient adrenally suppressed? Is it necessary to use stress doses of corticosteroids in the perioperative period?

Answers: The presence of adrenal suppression cannot be predicted in this patient on an intermediate dose of glucocorticoids. Additional testing or empirical coverage with stress-dose glucocorticoids is necessary.

Discussion: Surgery and anesthesia pose a physiologic stress that leads to an increase in endogenous levels of **adrenocorticotropic hormone (ACTH)** and serum cortisol. As a result, patients who take exogenous doses of glucocorticoids and may be potentially adrenally suppressed have a potential risk of clinically significant adrenal insufficiency in the perioperative period, usually manifesting as hypotension or tachycardia. Investigators first made these observations in a pair of case reports in the 1950s of two young patients who were taking long-term corticosteroids who died unexpectedly after routine orthopedic surgery. Since then, considerable debate has existed as to which patients taking exogenous glucocorticoids should be presumed to have adrenal suppression, which patients' adrenal axis should be studied, and which patients require perioperative stress doses of glucocorticoids. This debate has continued as a result of a relative paucity of clinical studies in the field. More recent studies suggest that previous dosage recommendations for glucocorticoid coverage were excessive and that fewer patients than previously believed require stress steroid coverage.

The benefit of perioperative stress doses of glucocorticoids in patients receiving long-term steroid therapy has been called into question. In one study, 18 patients taking long-term daily glucocorticoids (average daily dose of prednisone, 14 mg) were randomized to perioperative intravenous treatment with stress doses of hydrocortisone or placebo in addition to their usual prednisone doses. All patients had a blunted response to preoperative ACTH stimulation testing and had potential suppression of the pituitary adrenal axis. One patient in each group had perioperative hypotension that responded to intravenous fluids only. The authors concluded that patients receiving low-dose to intermediate-dose, long-term daily glucocorticoid therapy could undergo surgery safely when given their usual daily steroid dose without the need for stress dosing.

In another study, authors evaluated a cohort of 52 renal transplant patients who were taking long-term daily glucocorticoid therapy (average doses of prednisone, 5 to 15 mg daily). When undergoing a variety of minor and major surgical procedures, these patients received only their usual daily prednisone dose without stress-dose coverage. There were no cases of adrenal insufficiency in the perioperative period as determined clinically or by 24-hour urinary cortisol levels. The authors concluded that ACTH stimulation testing to determine which patients would require perioperative stress steroid coverage was overly sensitive and would result in treating more patients than necessary.

High-potency topical steroids applied to large portions of the body surface may cause biochemically apparent adrenal axis suppression. Likewise, long-term use of high doses of inhaled corticosteroids for the treatment of asthma cause suppression of the pituitary adrenal axis. Although adrenal suppression may be detected in each of these cases, most authors do not recommend prophylactic use of perioperative stress-dose steroids for such patients. Rather the clinician should be alert to this possibility and be prepared to use stress-dose steroids in the perioperative period if clinical suspicion of adrenal insufficiency exists (e.g., hypotension that is unresponsive to intravenous fluids).

It is now apparent that not all patients who take long-term daily glucocorticoids or who have taken them in the recent past are at risk for clinically significant adrenal insufficiency in the perioperative period. Patients who have received any dose of glucocorticoid for <3 weeks and those who take daily doses of <5 mg/d of prednisone or its equivalent are not adrenally suppressed and do not require supplemental stress dosing of steroids. Patients taking >20 mg/d of prednisone or its equivalent for >3 weeks should be considered to have adrenal suppression. Likewise, any patient taking such a dose within the previous 6 months is at risk for adrenal axis suppression.

Patients taking intermediate doses of daily steroids may or may not have adrenal suppression. For these patients, the clinician routinely can administer stress doses of perioperative steroids or, if time allows in elective surgery, study the pituitary adrenal axis by ACTH stimulation testing. Although many protocols exist for ACTH stimulation testing, a cortisol value of ≥ 18 µg/dL at any time (baseline or any time after ACTH administration) indicates normal adrenal function and predicts no need for supplemental perioperative stress steroid coverage.

More recent recommendations for perioperative steroid management take into account the severity of the surgical stress. For patients undergoing minor surgery (e.g., inguinal hernia repair under local anesthesia), patients may take their usual daily dose of glucocorticoids without supplementation. For moderate surgical stress, patients can be given 50 mg of hydrocortisone intravenously before surgery and 25 mg intravenously every 8 hours for 24 hours, then resume their usual dose. For major surgical stress, the clinician can give 100 mg of hydrocortisone intravenously before surgery and 50 mg intravenously every 8 hours for 24 hours, then taper the dose by half each day until resumption of usual daily dose.

The present patient took an intermediate daily dose of glucocorticoids (5 to 20 mg of prednisone per day). Her likelihood of having adrenal axis suppression also was intermediate. Because this surgery is elective, the clinician could study adrenal function with an ACTH stimulation test or could choose to use perioperative stress steroid coverage empirically. In the latter case, the following regimen is recommended: 50 mg of hydrocortisone intravenously before surgery, 25 mg intravenously every 8 hours for 24 hours, then resume usual dose the next day for moderate-risk surgery.

Clinical Pearls

1. Any patient taking >20 mg of prednisone daily for at least 3 weeks at any time in the past 6 months should be considered to have pituitary adrenal axis suppression.

2. Patients taking <5 mg of prednisone per day may proceed to surgery without stress steroid coverage.

3. Patients taking intermediate doses of daily glucocorticoids are candidates for either ACTH stimulation testing of pituitary adrenal function or empirical stress steroid coverage.

4. Dose schedules for stress steroid coverage depend on the magnitude of the surgical stress for the particular procedure.

5. The clinician should be alert to the possibility of adrenal insufficiency in any patient taking daily glucocorticoids if perioperative hypotension develops that is unresponsive to intravenous fluids.

REFERENCES

1. Salem M, Tainsh RE, Bromberg J, et al: Perioperative glucocorticoid coverage: A reassessment 42 years after emergence of a problem. Ann Surg 219:416–425, 1994.
2. Bromberg JS, Baliga P, Cofer JB, et al: Stress steroids are not required for patients receiving a renal allograft and undergoing operation. J Am Coll Surg 180:532–536, 1995.
3. Glowniak JV, Loriaux DL: A double-blind study of perioperative steroid requirements in secondary adrenal insufficiency. Surgery 121:123–129, 1997.
4. Lipworth BJ: Systemic adverse effects of inhaled corticosteroid therapy: A systematic review and meta-analysis. Arch Intern Med 159:941–955, 1999.
5. Welsh GA, Manzullo E, Orth DN: The surgical patient taking corticosteroids. In Rose BD (ed): UpToDate. Wellesley, UpToDate, 2001.

PATIENT 24

A 62-year-old man with hypertension in the postanesthesia care unit after elective total hip replacement

A 62-year-old man is seen in the postanesthesia care unit 1 hour after elective total hip replacement for degenerative arthritis and daily pain. He has a 10-year history of well-controlled hypertension. His blood pressure immediately before induction of anesthesia was 138/86 mmHg. He had an uneventful intraoperative course that included no significant swings in blood pressure. The anesthesiologists have requested a medical consultation because of the new development of a blood pressure of 180/110 mmHg 1 hour after completion of surgery. The patient reports significant incisional pain but denies chest pain or shortness of breath. He took his usual morning doses of antihypertensive medication on the day of surgery. Past medical history also includes gastroesophageal reflux disease. Outpatient medications are atenolol, 50 mg daily; hydrochlorothiazide, 25 mg daily; lisinopril, 20 mg daily; and ranitidine, 150 mg twice daily.

Physical Examination: Temperature 99.6°F, blood pressure 180/110, heart rate 108, respirations 16, oxygen saturation 96% on 2 L/min nasal prongs. General appearance: Uncomfortable appearing but in no acute respiratory distress. Chest: clear. Cardiac: tachycardic $S_1S_2S_4$, no murmurs. Jugular venous pressure 6 cm. Extremities: tense hematoma beneath hip incision.

Laboratory Findings: Hct 30%, WBC 13,400/μL. ECG: sinus tachycardia but otherwise normal.

Questions: What is the cause of this patient's hypertension? How should it be treated?

Answers: Postoperative pain. Adequate analgesia and intravenous antihypertensive agents are the principal treatment strategies.

Discussion: Significant postoperative hypertension (blood pressure >190/100 mmHg) occurs in approximately 3% of unselected patients undergoing general surgery. The mechanism of this acute rise in blood pressure after surgery is unknown. A previous history of hypertension is the most important risk factor. In an early large study of 1844 patients, 60 patients developed postoperative hypertension; 60% of these patients had a history of hypertension. The elevated blood pressure usually began within 30 minutes of the end of the operation and typically lasted 2 hours. Complications occurred only in patients whose hypertension lasted for >2 hours after surgery. Other contributing factors in this cohort were pain (36%), excitement on emergence from anesthesia (16%), hypoxia (17%), and reaction to endotracheal tube (15%).

Patients are more likely to develop postoperative hypertension after certain types of surgery. In Goldman's early work, postoperative hypertension occurred most commonly after abdominal aortic aneurysm surgery (57% of patients), peripheral vascular surgery (29%), and intraperitoneal or intrathoracic surgeries (8%). Only 4% of patients undergoing all other types of surgery developed postoperative hypertension. Other reports have identified a high incidence of postoperative hypertension among patients undergoing aortic valve and carotid artery surgery.

When postoperative hypertension occurs, the first priority is to identify and treat precipitating factors. Most important among these is **pain**. Frequently, adequate analgesia, such as intravenous morphine or fentanyl, normalizes the blood pressure. When a remediable cause for pain is present, it should be treated. Examples include traction on the surgical wound or bladder catheter. Another important cause is bladder distention in the supine postoperative patient who may have received intravenous narcotics as part of the anesthetic management. Other factors that may contribute to postoperative hypertension include agitation, hypoxia, hypercarbia, and volume expansion. Clinicians should search systematically for the presence of these factors and treat as appropriate.

When remediable factors have been excluded, attention turns to treatment of persistent substantial blood pressure elevations so as to minimize morbidity. The goal is to reduce blood pressure to the high-normal range (140/90 mmHg) but not lower. Intravenous formulations are available for most of the commonly used classes of antihypertensive agents and are preferred, given the need for urgent reduction in blood pressure, variable absorption of oral medications in the immediate postoperative period, and difficulty administering oral medications to patients who have not awoken completely after anesthesia.

All long-term oral medications should have been given to the patient up to and including the morning of surgery. If this was not the case and the outpatient regimen includes a β-blocker, drug selection for the treatment of postoperative hypertension must take this into account. In this case, β-blocker withdrawal may precipitate hypertension and myocardial ischemia. The treatment of choice would be an intravenous β-blocker, such as propranolol, esmolol, or labetalol. Likewise, abrupt withdrawal of clonidine may cause rebound hypertension. For patients previously taking clonidine that was abruptly withdrawn, intravenous methyldopa or labetalol or a clonidine patch is appropriate therapy for postoperative hypertension.

In all other cases, clinicians need not select the particular intravenous agent based on the patient's long-term daily medications. Because catecholamine responses to surgery may contribute to the development of postoperative hypertension, it is reasonable first to use an intravenous β-blocker if no contraindication to its use exists. The clinician may administer any of the parenteral drugs used for the treatment of hypertensive emergencies, however, including intravenous nitroprusside, hydralazine, enalaprilat, and nicardipine, in addition to the β-blockers mentioned earlier. Sublingual nifedipine should not be used for the treatment of postoperative hypertension because of reports of myocardial ischemia, stroke, and other complications among patients so treated with hypertensive urgencies.

In the present patient, pain from a wound hematoma was a contributing factor to his postoperative pain. The surgical team should evaluate the need for drainage of the hematoma or revision of the incision. Intravenous narcotics, such as morphine or fentanyl, should be used to provide adequate pain relief. If significant blood pressure elevations persist, an intravenous β-blocker should be used to reduce blood pressure to approximately 140/90 mmHg.

Clinical Pearls

1. A preoperative history of hypertension is the most important risk factor for postoperative hypertension.

2. Severe elevations of postoperative blood pressure in the first 2 hours after surgery are most common among patients undergoing aortic aneurysm, peripheral vascular, and carotid surgeries.

3. When postoperative hypertension develops, the clinician first should search for and treat remediable causes, such as pain, hypoxia, hypercarbia, bladder distention, and volume expansion.

4. If postoperative hypertension persists after treatment of remediable factors, intravenous agents, particularly intravenous β-blockers, should be used to lower blood pressure to 140/90 mmHg.

REFERENCES

1. Gal TJ, Cooperman LH: Hypertension in the immediate postoperative period. Br J Anaesth 47:70–72, 1975.
2. Goldman L, Caldera DL: Risks of general anesthesia and elective operation in the hypertensive patient. Anesthesiology 50:285–292, 1979.
3. Grossman E, Messerli FH, Grodzicki T, Kowey P: Should a moratorium be placed on sublingual nifedipine capsules given for hypertensive emergencies and pseudoemergencies? JAMA 276:1328–1331, 1996.
4. Levy JH: Treatment of perioperative hypertension. Anesthesiol Clin North Am 17:567–579, 1999.

PATIENT 25

A 64-year-old woman with a productive cough preparing for elective hemicolectomy

A 64-year-old woman presents to the preoperative medical evaluation clinic before hemicolectomy. One month earlier, in evaluation of iron-deficiency anemia, she was found to have a cecal mass, which biopsy confirmed to be an adenocarcinoma. Her past medical history is otherwise benign. Five days ago, she developed a runny nose, sore throat, and a cough productive of yellow-to-green mucus. She has had low-grade fevers (≤99.6°F). She is otherwise well. She takes no regular medications.

Physical Examination: Temperature 99.4°F, blood pressure 140/82, heart rate 80, respirations 14, oxygen saturation on room air 98%. HEENT: oropharynx normal without injection, no sinus tenderness. No lymphadenopathy. Chest: no wheezes, rhonchi, or rales. Cardiac: normal S_1S_2, no murmurs, rubs, gallops, or jugular venous distention.

Laboratory Findings: Hct 38%, WBC 8600/μL. Chest radiograph: see Figure.

Question: Can this patient proceed to surgery without delay?

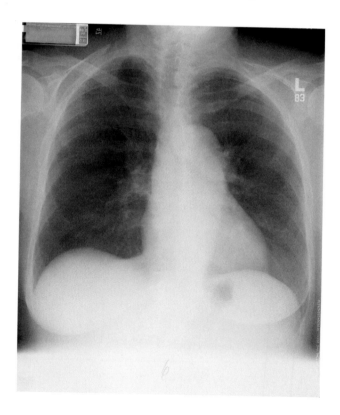

Answer: Delay elective surgery in the presence of respiratory infection.

Discussion: The risk factors for postoperative pulmonary complications are well established. Most important are the surgical site, duration of surgery, type of anesthetic, presence of chronic obstructive pulmonary disease, and smoking history. Upper abdominal surgery, such as hemicolectomy in this patient, carries the greatest risk. The contribution of respiratory infection to risk of postoperative pulmonary complications is less well understood. The principal mechanism contributing to pulmonary complications is a decrease in lung volume that may lead to atelectasis, mucus plugging, and pneumonia. It seems intuitive that other factors that may add to this mechanism, such as untreated respiratory infection, would increase risk further. This possibility has not been well studied, however.

A few studies evaluating the risk of pulmonary complications among patients who already are at low risk exist. One report found no increase in risk among children undergoing myringotomy who had an active upper respiratory tract infection compared with children who did not have such an infection. No studies have evaluated systematically the impact of upper respiratory tract infection on postoperative pulmonary complication rates in adults undergoing high-risk surgery.

In contrast, patients with active lower respiratory tract infection already may be at higher risk for complications resulting from airway reactivity and preexisting mucus production that may contribute to the development of atelectasis and parenchymal infection; this was suggested by a study in which the authors obtained routine tracheal aspirates immediately after intubation for cardiac surgery. Only 1.4% of patients with negative tracheal aspirates developed postoperative lower respiratory tract infection, whereas 31% of patients with positive aspirates developed postoperative pneumonia. Although the patients with positive tracheal aspirates did not have a clinically apparent bronchitis before surgery, this study supports a physiologic plausibility that airway infec-

tion, such as bronchitis, may predispose to postoperative pneumonia.

Studies evaluating the risk posed by respiratory infection are confounded by the difficulty in establishing a diagnosis of infection and the lack of a consistent reference standard. Symptoms of allergic rhinitis, asthma, bacterial bronchitis, and viral respiratory infection overlap sufficiently that diagnoses based on history taking may include patients without actual respiratory infection.

Many studies have shown that the indiscriminate routine use of preoperative antibiotics does not reduce the risk of postoperative pulmonary complications. The appropriate use of antibiotics to treat respiratory infection, as part of a comprehensive regimen for high-risk patients, does reduce risk.

The studies in this area are few and of variable quality. It is not possible to construct an evidence-based approach to the patient preparing for surgery with suspected respiratory infection. In truly elective surgery, delay of surgery is inconvenient but does not add risk. Using the principle of "do no harm," it is reasonable to delay elective surgery in the presence of respiratory infection until the infection has run its course or been treated appropriately. Upper respiratory infection probably poses less risk than lower respiratory infection, but few data exist regarding this question. Lower respiratory infection is suggested by the new development of a cough with purulent sputum or a change in the character or quantity of sputum in a patient with chronic cough. In this case, it is appropriate to use antibiotics to treat lower respiratory infection before proceeding to nonemergent surgery.

In the present patient, symptoms suggested upper respiratory infection with possible superimposed bronchitis. Because the surgery was elective and a brief delay would not harm the patient, the surgery should be canceled and the bronchitis treated first.

Clinical Pearls

1. The risk of upper respiratory infection among adults undergoing surgery is unknown but probably is small.

2. Lower respiratory infection seems to increase the risk of postoperative pulmonary complications.

3. Elective surgery should be delayed in the presence of respiratory infection.

4. Lower respiratory tract bacterial infection should be treated with antibiotics before proceeding to surgery.

REFERENCES

1. Laszlo G, Archer GG, Darrell JH, et al: The diagnosis and prophylaxis of pulmonary complications of surgical operation. Br J Surg 60:129–134, 1973.
2. Tait AR, Knight PR: The effects of general anesthesia on upper respiratory tract infections in children. Anesthesiology 67:930–935, 1987.
3. Fennelly ME, Hall GM: Anaesthesia and upper respiratory tract infections: A non-existent hazard? (editorial). Br J Anaesth 64:535–536, 1990.
4. Carrel T, Schmid ER, von Segesser L, et al: Preoperative assessment of the likelihood of infection of the lower respiratory tract after cardiac surgery. Thorac Cardiovasc Surgeon 39:85–88, 1991.

PATIENT 26

A 54-year-old woman with morbid obesity preparing for cholecystectomy

A 54-year-old woman has a history of biliary colic and is scheduled for elective laparoscopic cholecystectomy. She presents to the preoperative testing center before elective surgery. Her medical history includes morbid obesity, and recent weights have ranged from 300 to 350 lb. She has well-controlled hypertension and low back pain. Medications include lisinopril and hydrochlorothiazide.

Physical Examination: Blood pressure 140/88, heart rate 76, respirations 14. Weight 334 lb. General appearance: Obese but otherwise well-appearing woman in no distress. Chest: clear. Cardiac: normal S_1S_2 with S_4 but no S_3, murmur, or rub. Jugular venous pressure is normal. Abdomen: obese, soft, nontender, without masses or hepatosplenomegaly. Extremities: trace pitting edema bilaterally to the midcalf.

Laboratory Findings: CBC normal. Liver function tests normal. Electrolytes, BUN, creatinine normal. ECG: normal sinus rhythm at 70, normal intervals and axis, left ventricular hypertrophy but otherwise normal morphology.

Question: How does morbid obesity influence perioperative morbidity and mortality?

Answer: With the exception of a higher incidence of wound infections, morbid obesity is not a significant risk factor for major adverse perioperative outcomes.

Discussion: It seems intuitive that obesity would increase the risk of perioperative complications and adverse outcomes. The data suggest, however, that morbid obesity does not confer additional risk for major adverse postoperative outcomes. The areas of potential interest include cardiac, pulmonary, and infectious complications.

Since the first multifactorial cardiac risk index by Goldman et al in 1977, several risk indices and cardiac risk stratification guidelines have been published. None of these indices has identified obesity as an independent predictor of postoperative cardiac complications or cardiac death; this includes the original Goldman index, the Detsky modified cardiac risk index, the Lee revised cardiac risk index, the American College of Cardiology guideline for perioperative cardiovascular evaluation, and the American College of Physicians guideline for the assessment of cardiac risk. This risk stratification applies to all major general surgery. Studies that have used clinical criteria to predict risk in major vascular surgery also have failed to identify obesity as a risk factor for postoperative cardiac complications. Although this may seem counterintuitive, as obesity is a risk factor for coronary artery disease, this observation has been consistent over multiple studies and is beyond debate. Clinicians should not deny or modify surgery because of fear of cardiac risk related to obesity alone.

The relationship between obesity and postoperative pulmonary complications is more controversial. Obesity reduces functional residual capacity, total lung capacity, and vital capacity by 30%. The work of breathing also increases because of the heavier chest wall and abnormal diaphragm position. Given that decreased lung volumes after surgery are the major physiologic substrate for the development of postoperative pulmonary complication, one might expect an increase in pulmonary complication rates for obese surgical patients. Most studies have not shown such a relationship, however.

Multiple reports that include different major surgical procedures generally have shown no increase in pulmonary complication rates for obese patients. In a report of adverse outcomes after coronary artery bypass graft surgery in 2299 patients, no difference existed in the rates of prolonged mechanical ventilation or pneumonia between obese and nonobese patients. There was a nonsignificant trend toward lower complication rates in the obese patients. Two studies of the role of obesity in complications after laparoscopic cholecystectomy have shown no difference in overall mortality or pulmonary complications. Likewise, studies have shown no difference in pulmonary complication rates between obese and nonobese patients undergoing total hip replacement. In a review of previous reports, the overall incidence of postoperative pulmonary complications among general surgical patients was 21% for obese and nonobese patients.

A related issue is that of obstructive sleep apnea. Obesity is the principal risk factor for obstructive sleep apnea, and some obese surgical patients have previously unrecognized sleep apnea. The presence of obstructive sleep apnea increases the likelihood of airway management problems in the immediate postoperative period, such as the need for reintubation because of upper airway dysfunction and postoperative oxygen desaturation. Sleep apnea by itself has not been shown to increase the risk of important postoperative pulmonary complications, such as pneumonia, atelectasis, or respiratory failure. Anesthesiologists should be aware of the possibility of postoperative airway management problems in the morbidly obese patient, but consulting internists should not conclude that unrecognized sleep apnea increases the risk for postoperative pulmonary complications.

In contrast to pulmonary and cardiac complications, there is an increase in the risk of surgical wound infections among obese patients. Obese patients have a twofold increase in the risk of wound infections in general surgery and of sternal wound infections in coronary artery bypass surgery. The relative risk attributed to obesity is not as great, however, as that seen among patients with diabetes; obesity is a less powerful risk factor for wound infections.

In the present patient, the history of morbid obesity increased the risk of postoperative wound infection, an issue primarily in the domain of the surgeon. She had no increased risk of mortality or postoperative cardiac or pulmonary complications. She required no additional preoperative evaluation or risk stratification.

Clinical Pearls

1. Morbid obesity does not increase perioperative mortality.
2. Obesity confers a twofold increase in the risk of wound infection.
3. Obesity is not a risk factor for postoperative cardiac complications.
4. Clinicians should not deny major surgery based on the presence of morbid obesity alone.

REFERENCES

1. Phillips EH, Carroll BJ, Fallas MJ, Pearlstein AR: Comparison of laparoscopic cholecystectomy in obese and non-obese patients. Am Surgeon 60:316–321, 1994.
2. Birkmeyer NJ, Charlesworth DC, Hernandez F, et al: Obesity and risk of adverse outcomes associated with coronary bypass surgery. 97:1689–1694, 1998.
3. Flancbaum L, Choban PS: Surgical implications of obesity. Annu Rev Med 49:215–234, 1998.
4. Gatsoulis N, Koulas S, Kiparos G, et al: Laparoscopic cholecystectomy in obese and nonobese patients. Obes Surg 9:459–461, 1999.
5. Smetana GW: Preoperative pulmonary evaluation. N Engl J Med 340:937–944, 1999.

PATIENT 27

A 73-year-old man with atrial fibrillation after coronary artery bypass surgery

A 73-year-old man has a history of progressive exertional angina that has limited his lifestyle despite maximal antianginal medical therapy. On cardiac catheterization, he was found to have significant three-vessel coronary artery disease with preserved left ventricular function. Two days ago, he underwent uneventful three-vessel coronary artery bypass surgery. Today, on postoperative day 2, he develops palpitations and is found to be in atrial fibrillation with a rate of 110 beats/min. Blood pressure is stable; he has had no congestive heart failure. Past medical history includes elevated cholesterol and hypertension. Medications at the time of admission included atenolol, atorvastatin, and aspirin.

Physical Examination: Temperature 98.2°F, blood pressure 112/66, heart rate 110 and irregularly irregular, respirations 14. General appearance: Well-appearing man with pulmonary artery catheter in right internal jugular vein, extubated, and speaking comfortably. Chest: dullness at left base with tubular breath sounds and crackles a quarter of the way up. Right chest clear. Cardiac: irregular rhythm, normal S_1S_2, II/VI systolic ejection murmur at left upper sternal border. Jugular venous pressure flat. Extremities: no edema.

Laboratory Findings: Hct 31%, WBC 8600/μL. Electrolytes, BUN, creatinine normal. Chest radiograph: left lower lobe partial atelectasis. ECG: see Figure (next page).

Questions: What are the risk factors for postoperative arrhythmia? How can this be prevented?

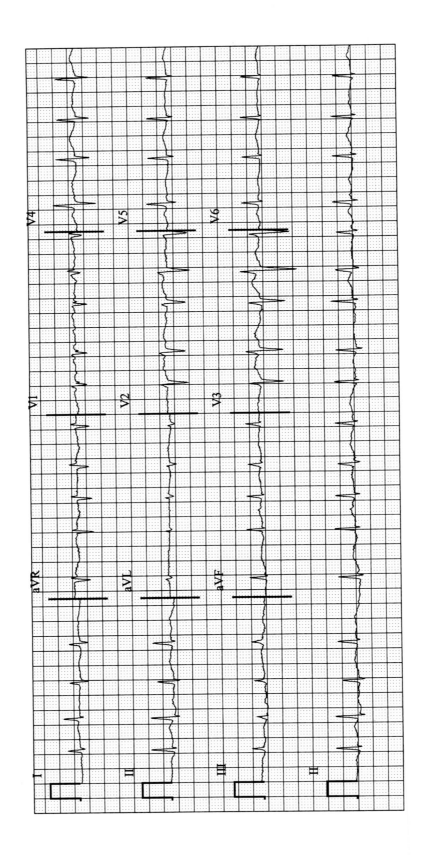

Answer: Age >70 years, valvular heart disease, hypertension, left atrial enlargement, and hypokalemia. β-blockers may reduce this risk.

Discussion: A history of preoperative arrhythmia is only a minor risk factor for the development of important postoperative cardiac complications, such as postoperative myocardial infarction or cardiac death. In the original Goldman and modified Detsky cardiac risk indices, rhythms other than sinus and atrial or ventricular ectopy were each minor risk factors in multivariate analyses. The revised cardiac risk index of Lee, which outperforms the original indices, does not include preoperative arrhythmia as a significant risk factor.

Postoperative arrhythmias usually are not a cause of significant morbidity. These are most commonly atrial arrhythmias; atrial fibrillation is most common. Several preoperative risk factors identify patients at high risk for postoperative arrhythmia, particularly atrial fibrillation. Preoperative hypokalemia predicts the need for cardiopulmonary resuscitation and the likelihood of perioperative arrhythmia in cardiac surgery patients. In particular, serum potassium <3.5 mmol/L predicted risk. Among patients undergoing cardiac bypass surgery, risk factors include age >70 years, valvular heart disease, hypertension, and left ventricular dysfunction. Left atrial enlargement, sepsis, and a previous history of atrial fibrillation are additional risk factors. Age is the most important risk factor. The risk of postoperative atrial fibrillation after cardiothoracic surgery is 5% for patients <40 years of age but 30% for patients >70 years.

The incidence of arrhythmia varies considerably depending on the type of surgery. In a classic early report of patients undergoing noncardiac surgery, the overall incidence of postoperative arrhythmia was 4%. In contrast, postoperative atrial arrhythmias occur in 10% of patients undergoing lung resection, 40% of patients undergoing coronary bypass surgery, and 50% of patients undergoing valvular surgery. Arrhythmia most commonly occurs within 4 days after surgery.

In patients at risk, perioperative mechanisms that contribute to the development of arrhythmia include hypoxia, hypercarbia, myocardial ischemia, catecholamine release, electrolyte abnormalities, and medications. In the instance of cardiac surgery, additional specific factors include atrial distention, surgical trauma to atria, and mechanical pericarditis. Several studies have shown that perioperative β-blockers reduce the risk for postoperative atrial arrhythmias. Conventional antiarrhythmic drugs, such as quinidine and procainamide, do not seem to reduce the risk of postoperative atrial arrhythmias. In patients who are taking β-blockers preoperatively, the inadvertent abrupt withdrawal of these drugs leads to a particularly high risk of postoperative arrhythmia.

The approach to treatment of postoperative atrial arrhythmias is similar to that in the nonsurgical period. Goals are the prevention of thromboembolic complications through anticoagulation in the case of atrial fibrillation, rate control, and conversion to sinus rhythm. Uniquely in the postoperative setting, additional factors may contribute to the risk of arrhythmia, including volume overload, pain, anemia, and atelectasis or pneumonia, particularly involving the lingula. When present, these factors should be treated and optimized.

The present patient underwent coronary artery bypass surgery, a procedure that carries a high risk of postoperative atrial arrhythmia. His age and a history of hypertension were risk factors. Continuation of his preoperative β-blockers and the use of intravenous β-blockers in the immediate perioperative period would reduce his risk of postoperative atrial fibrillation. If preoperative hypokalemia was present, it should have been corrected before surgery. The treatment of atrial fibrillation was similar to that in the nonsurgical setting.

Clinical Pearls

1. Atrial tachyarrhythmias, particularly atrial fibrillation, are the most common postoperative arrhythmias.

2. Cardiac valvular surgery, coronary artery bypass surgery, and lung resection carry the highest risk of postoperative arrhythmia.

3. Advanced age, a history of atrial fibrillation, left ventricular dysfunction, preoperative hypokalemia, and hypertension are risk factors for the development of postoperative arrhythmia.

4. The treatment of postoperative atrial arrhythmias is the same as treatment in the nonoperative setting. Goals include rate control, maintenance of sinus rhythm, and anticoagulation for atrial fibrillation to prevent thromboembolic complications.

REFERENCES

1. Goldman L: Supraventricular tachyarrhythmias in hospitalized adults after surgery: Clinical correlates in patients over 40 years of age after major noncardiac surgery. Chest 73:450–454, 1978.
2. Ommen SR, Odell JA, Stanton MS: Atrial arrhythmias after cardiothoracic surgery. N Engl J Med 336:1429–1434, 1997.
3. Dyszkiewicz W, Skrzypczak M: Atrial fibrillation after surgery of the lung: Clinical analysis of risk factors. Eur J Cardiothorac Surg 13:625–628, 1998.
4. Bayliff CD, Massel DR, Inculet RI, et al: Propranolol for the prevention of postoperative arrhythmias in general thoracic surgery. Ann Thorac Surg 67:182–186, 1999.
5. Wahr JA, Parks R, Boisvert D, et al: Preoperative serum potassium levels and perioperative outcomes in cardiac surgery patients. JAMA 281:2203–2210, 1999.
6. Zama AG, Archbold A, Helft G, et al: Atrial fibrillation after coronary artery bypass surgery: A model for preoperative risk stratification. Circulation 101:1403–1408, 2000.

PATIENT 28

A 42-year-old man with hypertension, headaches, and flushing

A 42-year-old man with hypertension, headaches, and flushing presents for elective hernia repair. During the preoperative evaluation of his poorly controlled hypertension, he is found to have an adrenal mass. Studies on 24-hour urine collection confirm elevated catecholamines. He is now scheduled for tumor removal. He has a history of poorly controlled hypertension but has no chest pain or shortness of breath.

Physical Examination: Pulse 94; respiratory rate 14; blood pressure 178/94. Skin: no lesions. HEENT: normal. Chest: lungs clear to auscultation, no wheezing or rales. Cardiac: regular rhythm, no murmurs, gallops, or rubs appreciated. Abdomen: no masses palpated, no abdominal bruits, no organomegaly, no tenderness, normal active bowel sounds. Extremities: no cyanosis, clubbing, or edema. Neurologic: awake, oriented, no focal deficits.

Laboratory Findings: CBC normal. Blood chemistry normal. Thyroid function tests normal. 24-hour urine: elevations in vanillylmandelic acid and metanephrines. ECG: normal sinus rhythm, left ventricular hypertrophy by voltage, no ischemic changes. Chest radiograph: no acute infiltrate. Computed tomography scan of abdomen: 3-cm adrenal mass.

Question: What recommendations should be made concerning the patient's preoperative medications?

Answer: Preoperative blood pressure control should be achieved by titrating phenoxybenzamine, which is a nonspecific, long-acting α-blocker.

Discussion: Although high blood pressure is common, it is only in rare cases (<0.2%) that the blood pressure elevation can be attributed to **pheochromocytoma**. The classic presentation includes a triad of symptoms: episodic headache, sweating, and tachycardia. Only half of patients with pheochromocytoma have paroxysms of high blood pressure; in most, the more common presentation is of what appears to be essential hypertension. Less common associations include dilated cardiomyopathy, orthostatic hypotension, and either pallor or flushing. Most symptoms are thought to be related to the hypersecretion of norepinephrine or epinephrine or both from the tumor.

Treatment is surgical resection. Preoperative preparation of the patient is aimed at controlling blood pressure and heart rate. Traditionally, patients are premedicated with phenoxybenzamine, 20 mg once a day, with increases in doses every few days until the blood pressure is brought under control. β-Blockers can be added later to help control heart rate. (Never start the β-blocker first: unopposed α-receptor stimulation in the company of β blockade would lead to a further increase in blood pressure.) These preoperative medicines should be administered for at least 14 days to optimize the patient for surgery.

A newer approach to preoperative preparation has been studied in a small group of patients. These patients all were premedicated with volume expansion, but they did not receive additional blood pressure medicines if their blood pressure was under control. If the blood pressure was elevated, the patients were given calcium channel blockers, which helped lessen coronary artery spasm and did not lead to orthostatic hypotension. Phenoxybenzamine was added only in a small subset of patients who still needed additional blood pressure control. The patients in this treatment group needed less intraoperative fluid replacement and had a lower incidence of complications.

The present patient had the traditional therapy of phenoxybenzamine started 2 weeks preoperatively. This agent was added to his usual regimen of enalapril, labetalol, and hydrochlorothiazide. He also received volume expansion preoperatively. His blood pressure remained fairly stable perioperatively. At the onset of surgery, blood pressure was 148/82 mmHg; peak blood pressure was 160/92 mmHg, and nadir was 116/54 mmHg.

Clinical Pearls

1. No universally accepted preoperative preparation for pheochromocytoma exists. Most treatments include phenoxybenzamine, 20 mg/d, until blood pressure and symptoms are under control. New regimens include pretreatment with calcium channel blockers.

2. Postoperative hypotension can be avoided by providing adequate fluid replacement preoperatively.

3. The clinician must be alert to hypoglycemia, which can occur in a relatively high percentage of patients when catecholamine suppression is removed.

REFERENCES

1. Suzuki A, Taguchi S, Wakayama S: Repeated postoperative hypoglycemia in a woman with multiple pheochromocytomas. Jpn J Anesthesiol 48:1014–1016, 1999.
2. Bogdonoff DL, Vance ML: Uncommon endocrine disorders. In Stone DJ, Bogdonoff DL, Leisure GS, et al (eds): Perioperative Care. St Louis, Mosby, 1998, pp 272–280.
3. Ulchaker JC, Goldfarb D, Bravo EL, Novick AC: Successful outcomes in pheochromocytoma surgery in the modern era. J Urol 161:764–767, 1999.

PATIENT 29

A 48-year-old woman with postoperative agitation and confusion

A 48-year-old woman develops agitation and confusion on postoperative day 3 after an uncomplicated total abdominal hysterectomy. She is unable to give any further history because of her confused state.

Physical Examination: Temperature 99°F, blood pressure 124/78, pulse 104, respirations 20. Skin: no lesions. Mucosa: no petechiae. HEENT: normal. Chest: rapid respirations, shallow breathing with no rhonchi or rales. Cardiac: regular tachycardia, no murmurs or gallops. Abdomen: slightly distended, decreased bowel sounds, tender to palpation diffusely, with mild guarding but no rebound, no masses. Extremities: no edema, no calf tenderness. Neurologic: awake, agitated, following commands but confused, oriented to person but not to place or time.

Laboratory Findings: Hct 32%, WBC 7600/μl. Blood chemistry: sodium 123 mEq/L, potassium 4.1 mEq/L, serum osmolality 230 mOsm/kg, glucose 128 mg/dL. ECG: sinus tachycardia with no change compared with previous ECG. Chest radiograph(portable): of poor quality secondary to patient noncompliance, but no acute infiltrate can be identified. ABG (room air): pH 7.43, $PaCO_2$ 32 mmHg, PaO_2 80 mmHg, oxygen saturation 91%.

Question: What is the most likely cause of the patient's confusion and tachycardia?

Answer: This patient has postoperative hyponatremia, which may be the cause of confusion and tachycardia, although at this point in the evaluation, there is also suspicion that pulmonary embolism (or fat embolism) may be contributing to the clinical picture. Further testing is needed.

Additional Tests Indicate: Urine osmolality is 500 mOsm/kg of water.

Discussion: Hyponatremia in the postoperative state is a relatively common occurrence. Causes include increased antidiuretic hormone secretion secondary to pain, anxiety, nausea, stress, fear, underlying disease, or the administration of drugs including diuretics or narcotics. When severe, hyponatremia can lead to brain demyelination and death, so rapid attention to the problem is imperative.

Postoperative hyponatremia seems to be more common in premenopausal women, especially those who have received hypotonic fluids. Outcomes of women with encephalopathy from the hyponatremia are significantly worse in the premenopausal versus postmenopausal state. The clinician must pay close attention to pain control (because pain can worsen syndrome of inappropriate antidiuretic hormone [SIADH]) and to choice of intravenous fluids and fluid rate. Younger women who complain of postoperative headaches or nausea need to have serum sodium levels checked quickly.

Therapy of hyponatremia depends on the underlying cause. The first determination is **serum osmolality**. In the perioperative state, most cases are in the hypotonic category (see Figure). The next determination is of fluid status, which sometimes is difficult to assess postoperatively when extensive fluid shifts are occurring.

Treatment of the hypovolemic hyponatremias involves appropriate replacement of lost fluids, controlling diarrhea or vomiting, and stopping all medications that may be contributing (i.e., diuretics and angiotensin-converting enzyme [ACE] inhibitors). Fluid choice and rate of treatment depend on the severity of hyponatremia and the time frame during which the problem developed. Correction needs to be rapid enough to halt any neurologic sequelae (i.e., seizures or confusion) but slow enough to avoid so rapid a correction that brain trauma occurs. Normal saline or half-normal saline can be used to replace lost volume. If adrenal insufficiency

HYPONATREMIA

Serum Osmolality

Normal (280–295 mOsm/kg)	Low (<280 mOsm/kg)	High (>295 mOsm/kg)
ISOTONIC HYPONATREMIA:	HYPOTONIC HYPONATREMIA:	HYPERTONIC HYPONATREMIA:
Hyperproteinemia Hyperlipidemia	**Check Volume Status**	Hyperglycemia Mannitol, sorbitol Radiocontrast dyes

Hypovolemic:		Euvolemic:	Hypervolemic (edematous states):
U_{NA} <10 mEq/L	U_{NA} >20 mEq/L		
Dehydration Vomiting Diarrhea	Diuretics ACE inhibitor Mineralocorticoid deficiency Nephropathy	SIADH Postoperative hyponatremia Hypothyroidism Drug reactions	Congestive heart failure Cirrhosis Nephrotic syndrome

is included in the differential diagnosis, empirical use of corticosteroids is in order.

Treatment of hypervolemic hyponatremias, or the *edematous states,* includes treating the underlying disorder of congestive heart failure, liver, or kidney disease appropriately. Finally, the treatment of the euvolemic hyponatremias involves a rapid correction with hypertonic saline only if central nervous system symptoms are present. Correction is limited to 1 mEq/L/h (or 25 mEq/L) within the first day. Usually correction is aimed at 1 to 2 mEq/L/h over the first 24 hours, with a goal serum sodium of 125 mEq/L within that time frame. Alternatively the goal can be one half of the deficit over 24 hours if the serum sodium level is not severely decreased. Therapy with 3% saline should be reserved for symptomatic patients. The addition of furosemide is needed to facilitate excretion of free water in excess of sodium.

In the asymptomatic patient, correction need not be so rapid. Treatment is fluid restriction of 1 to 1.5 L/d. A gradual increase in sodium should be seen in several days. In mild postoperative hyponatremia (i.e., serum sodium 132 to 134 mEq/L), the problem generally resolves slowly on its own but warrants watching to ensure worsening is not occurring.

In the present patient, 3% saline was initiated because she was symptomatic. Her serum sodium was increased to 130 mEq/L over the first 24 hours, and her symptoms resolved. After that, she was treated with a moderate fluid restriction.

Clinical Pearls

1. In the postoperative patient with tachycardia or confusion, the clinician should consider electrolyte disorders and look for hyponatremia.

2. The clinician should check urine electrolytes and urine osmolality to confirm a diagnosis of SIADH-induced hyponatremia.

3. Postoperative hyponatremia can be severe in premenopausal women; a high index of suspicion should be maintained.

REFERENCES

1. Arieff AI: Hyponatremia, convulsions, respiratory arrest, and permanent brain damage after elective surgery in healthy woman. N Engl J Med 314:1529–1535, 1986.
2. Lauriat SM: The hyponatremic patient: Practical focus on therapy. J Am Soc Nephrol 8:1599–1607, 1997.
3. Gowrishanakar SH, et al: Acute hyponatremia in perioperative period: Insights into its pathophysiology and recommendations for management. Clin Nephrol 50:352–360, 1998.
4. Okuda T, et al: Fluid and electrolyte disorders. Current Medical Diagnosis and Treatment. 1999, pp 838–844.
5. Adrogue H, Maidas NE: Primary care: Hyponatremia. N Engl J Med Vol 342:1581–1589, 2000.

PATIENT 30

A 45-year-old man with recent deep venous thrombosis and new lower extremity fractures

A 45-year-old man injured in a motor vehicle accident is brought to the emergency department. He is diagnosed as having multiple fractures of the legs and pelvis. One month prior, he was hospitalized and treated for a deep venous thrombosis (DVT) in the right thigh. He denies any other medical problems; does not smoke cigarettes or drink alcohol; and is on warfarin, 7.5 mg/d. He denies chest pain, shortness of breath, or history of bleeding problems. Surgery to repair the femoral fractures is planned.

Physical Examination: Temperature 98°F, pulse 92, respirations 18, blood pressure 110/70. Heart: normal S_1 and S_2, no murmur or gallop. Chest: clear lungs. Extremities: no edema or calf tenderness, but multiple areas of tenderness and ecchymosis over both legs. The rest of the examination is normal.

Laboratory Findings: CBC: WBC 6200/μL, Hct 35%, platelets 90,000/μL. Blood chemistries normal. INR 2.0. Chest radiograph and ECG are normal.

Question: What would you recommend for DVT prophylaxis?

Answer: Although trauma patients are generally best treated with low-molecular-weight heparin, this patient is at very high risk for DVT recurrence and for PE, but must have anticoagulation reversal for surgery.

Discussion: This is a patient at high risk for developing a new DVT based on his past history of DVT, multiple lower extremity fractures, and presumed immobility over the next few weeks. The main issue is, however, that he had a DVT 1 month prior and requires full-dose anticoagulation for at least 6 months. The problem is that with his fractures and planned surgical procedures, he cannot be fully anticoagulated and undergo surgery. An inferior vena cava (IVC) filter may prevent any large lower extremity thrombi from becoming pulmonary emboli. The standard DVT prophylaxis in this case would be either low-molecular-weight heparin or warfarin. Technically, it would have been difficult (and contraindicated) to use intermittent pneumatic compression.

Anticoagulation can be resumed when the surgical team believes it is safe. The fact that the patient's platelet count is low may place him at even greater risk for bleeding. The cause of thrombocytopenia may be related to heparin he received for treatment of DVT, in which case unfractionated heparin and low-molecular-weight heparin would be contraindicated. Alternatively, the platelet count could be falsely low (pseudothrombocytopenia) secondary to clumping. This could be ascertained easily by examining the peripheral smear or by repeating the platelet count in a sodium citrate tube. There is nothing in the history to suggest that the patient has a bleeding diathesis, and it is unlikely that he has idiopathic thrombocytopenic purpura or disseminated intravascular coagulation. He presents a management dilemma in that his INR needs to come down before placement of a filter or major orthopedic surgery. Although giving him fresh frozen plasma and vitamin K in this setting may increase his risk of forming clot, one must bring down the INR to a more tolerable level (<1.5) before placing the IVC filter. Because vitamin K has a prolonged action and may make it difficult to increase the INR appropriately postoperatively, use of fresh frozen plasma is indicated. For increased intraoperative bleeding, use of platelets also may be helpful. In general, platelets, at least 100,000/μL, are required for adequate hemostasis in major surgery, although it is unusual for major bleeding to occur as long as the platelet count remains $>$50,000/μL.

In the present patient, an IVC filter was placed so that his anticoagulation could be reversed perioperatively. Twenty-four hours postoperatively, anticoagulation was begun again, but his INR was not therapeutic for 4 days.

Clinical Pearls

1. Low-molecular-weight heparin is the initial prophylaxis of choice for trauma patients if there are no contraindications.
2. Heparin-induced thrombocytopenia often occurs after the patient leaves the hospital.
3. If bleeding is a problem, mechanical modalities are indicated.
4. An IVC filter is indicated if there is a DVT that normally would be treated with full-dose anticoagulation but this is contraindicated.

REFERENCES

1. Lundberg GD: Practice parameter for the use of fresh-frozen plasma, cryoprecipitate, and platelets. JAMA 271:777–781, 1994.
2. Gerts WH, Heit JA, Claggett GP, et al: Prevention of venous thromboembolism. Chest 119:132S–175S, 2001.

PATIENT 31

A 72-year-old man with coronary artery disease and chronic obstructive pulmonary disease undergoing surgery

A 72-year-old man is scheduled for an aortoiliac bypass for severe claudication. Past history includes chronic obstructive pulmonary disease (COPD), hypertension, and an old inferior wall myocardial infarction (MI) (5 years ago). He was last hospitalized 1 year ago for COPD. Current medications include nitrates, amlodipine, inhaled β-agonists and steroids, and ipratropium bromide. He denies chest pain but has exertional dyspnea and occasional wheezing. His exercise capacity is limited to one block because of leg cramps.

Physical Examination: Temperature 98.8°, pulse 94, respirations 20, blood pressure 140/80. No use of accessory muscles for breathing. Heart: normal S_1 and S_2, no murmur or gallop. Chest: bilateral expiratory wheezing. Extremities: no edema or calf tenderness but decreased distal pulses in both legs. The rest of the examination is normal.

Laboratory Findings: CBC: WBC 9200/μL, Hct 48%, platelets 390,000/μL. Blood chemistries: normal except bicarbonate 32. ABG on room air: pH 7.42, PO_2 65 mmHg, PCO_2 45 mmHg. Chest radiograph: hyperinflation. ECG: normal sinus rhythm with Q waves in II, III, AVF; evidence of left ventricular hypertrophy.

Question: What would you recommend for preoperative risk evaluation and perioperative management?

Diagnosis and Treatment: Patient with coronary artery disease and COPD requiring further workup to assess severity of coronary artery disease before high-risk surgery and requiring treatment of pulmonary disease.

Discussion: This is a patient at high risk for perioperative cardiopulmonary complications. The most current guidelines being used for preoperative cardiac risk stratification are those from the American College of Cardiology and from the American College of Physicians. The American College of Physicians guideline is purely evidence based and makes no recommendations in the absence of strong evidence; the American College of Cardiology guideline is primarily evidence based but gives expert consensus opinion when there is no definitive evidence. The American College of Cardiology and American College of Physicians guidelines also differ with respect to classification of surgical procedures and use of exercise capacity. Based on American College of Cardiology criteria, this patient has an intermediate clinical predictor (previous MI), has poor exercise capacity, and is scheduled for high-risk surgery. Based on American College of Physicians criteria, he has 10 points (Detsky's modified cardiac index), has two Eagle or Vanzetto criteria (age, old MI), and is scheduled for vascular surgery.

Both algorithms would recommend noninvasive cardiac testing preoperatively—the question is which test. Although there are more data on dipyridamole thallium imaging, dobutamine echocardiography has had similar results with respect to positive and negative predictive values (although nuclear studies are more sensitive and echocardiography is more specific). Usually, it is up to the consultant to decide which test to use based on his or her experience and the expertise of the nuclear medicine and echocardiography personnel.

In this case, there is a relative contraindication to dipyridamole because of the patient's bronchospasm. This is a side effect seen with dipyridamole that can be treated readily with aminophylline. Some centers consider patients with a history of COPD, asthma, or mild obstructive airway disease able to undergo dipyridamole thallium testing safely (with various protocols), but most physicians believe that a patient with significant wheezing should not undergo this form of testing. Dobutamine echocardiography may be a better choice in this case and can provide information on wall motion abnormalities, systolic function, and valvular disease. Any evidence of significant ischemia (reperfusion or wall motion abnormalities that are large or in more than one coronary artery distribution) probably should be followed up with coronary angiography. Also, in view of this patient's bronchospasm, he is not a good candidate for perioperative β-blockers. His left ventricular hypertrophy does not confer any additional significant risk and does not require workup. His pulmonary disease should be medically optimized before surgery.

The present patient received flunisolide (AeroBid), albuterol and ipratropium bromide (Atrovent) preoperatively to optimize his pulmonary status. He underwent dobutamine echocardiography to stratify his cardiac risk further. He was found to have a wall motion abnormality of the inferior wall only and a preserved left ventricular ejection fraction. He subsequently underwent successful surgery.

Clinical Pearls

1. The American College of Cardiology guideline recommends noninvasive cardiac testing for patients with intermediate clinical predictors (prior MI, mild angina, diabetes, compensated or previous congestive heart failure) scheduled for high-risk surgery, especially if they have limited exercise capacity.

2. The American College of Physicians guideline recommends noninvasive cardiac testing for patients with intermediate risk and two or more *low-risk variables* (age >70, history of angina, diabetes, Q waves on ECG or history of MI, history of ventricular ectopy or congestive heart failure) scheduled for vascular surgery.

3. Dipyridamole thallium imaging is relatively contraindicated in patients with severe COPD or bronchospasm; dobutamine echocardiography is preferable in these cases.

REFERENCES

1. American College of Cardiology/American Heart Association task force on practice guidelines: Guidelines for perioperative cardiovascular evaluation for noncardiac surgery. J Am Coll Cardiol 27:910–948, 1996.
2. American College of Physicians: Guidelines for assessing and managing the perioperative risk from coronary artery disease associated with major noncardiac surgery. Ann Intern Med 127:309–312, 1997.
3. Palda VA, Detsky AS: Perioperative assessment and management of risk from coronary artery disease. Ann Intern Med 127:313–328, 1997.

PATIENT 32

A 50-year-old man with a systolic click undergoing urologic surgery

A 50-year-old man is scheduled for a transurethral prostatectomy for benign prostatic hyperplasia. Past history includes hypertension but no other medical problems. He was never hospitalized and is taking a β-blocker. He denies chest pain, dyspnea, or palpitations. His exercise capacity is excellent, and he can walk 2 miles without symptoms.

Physical Examination: Temperature 98.6°F, pulse 66, respirations 14, blood pressure 130/80. Heart: normal S_1 and S_2, systolic click noted but no murmur or gallop appreciated. Chest: clear. Extremities: no edema or calf tenderness. The rest of the examination is normal.

Laboratory Findings: CBC: WBC 7200/μL, Hct 47%, platelets 330,000/μL. Blood chemistries normal. ECG: normal sinus rhythm, no abnormalities noted.

Question: Does this patient need endocarditis prophylaxis?

Diagnosis: Yes.

Discussion: In patients undergoing transurethral resection of the prostate, data have shown a rate of postoperative bacteremia of 0 to 11% and a rate of postoperative bacteriuria of 12% to 54% when preoperative urine is sterile. Although there are insufficient data to show that preoperative antibiotics decrease the rate of postoperative urinary tract infection, bacteremia, or sepsis, there is reason to use antibiotics for endocarditis prophylaxis for susceptible patients. This is a patient potentially at risk for developing endocarditis based on the click, his age, and gender.

The most recent American Heart Association guideline discusses the risks associated with mitral valve prolapse. Previously, only patients with a murmur of mitral regurgitation were believed to be at risk and require prophylaxis; however, a dilemma arose in terms of what to do with patients who had no murmur clinically but evidence of mitral regurgitation on echocardiogram, a murmur that was heard only intermittently, and a murmur that was heard only during maneuvers or pharmacologic testing. Currently, it is believed that patients with an isolated systolic click may be likely to have intermittent mitral regurgitation. This condition may be associated with mitral valve prolapse or myxomatous degeneration.

Patients with significant regurgitation are more likely to be older and male. The recommendations are that the presence of a click, especially in a man >45 years old, should warrant further evaluation of mitral valve structure and function or prophylaxis in the absence of echocardiographic information. Mitral valve prolapse is considered a moderate risk for endocarditis and does not warrant the older recommendation of ampicillin and gentamicin, which currently are indicated only for the high-risk subgroup (prosthetic valve, previous endocarditis, and complex cyanotic congenital heart disease).

In the present patient, an echocardiogram should be obtained. If an echocardiogram were not done, antibiotic prophylaxis with amoxicillin (2 g orally 1 hour before the procedure) or ampicillin (2 g intramuscularly or intravenously 30 minutes before surgery) is indicated.

Clinical Pearls

1. Patients who are male, are >45 years old, and have the presence of a click may have increased risk for developing intermittent mitral regurgitation and endocarditis.

2. The American Heart Association guideline recommends further investigation of patients with a click even in the absence of a murmur.

3. Antibiotic prophylaxis for gastrointestinal and genitourinary procedures is different based on whether the patient is at moderate or high risk. Oral amoxicillin alone now can be given to the moderate-risk group.

REFERENCES
1. Dajani AS, Taubert KA, Wilson W, et al: Prevention of bacterial endocarditis—Recommendations by the American Heart Association. JAMA 1997; 277:1794–1801.
2. Anonymous: Antimicrobial prophylaxis is surgery. Med Lett 1995; 37: 79–82.
3. Page CP, Bohnen JMA, Fletcher R, et al: Antimicrobial prophylaxis for surgical wounds: guidelines for clinical care. Arch Surg 1993; 128: 79–88.

PATIENT 33

A 25-year-old woman at 12 weeks' gestation with hyperglycemia

A 25-year-old woman, gravida 2, para 1, presents for her initial obstetrics visit at 12 weeks' gestation. Her medical history is notable for gestational diabetes during her last pregnancy. Her fasting glucose at the time of presentation was 130 mg/dL. Her mother and one sister have type 2 diabetes mellitus.

Physical Examination: Weight 221 lb, height 65 inches. HEENT: normal. Chest: normal. Heart: normal. Abdomen: soft, nontender. Gestational age based on last menstrual period: 12 weeks and 4 days.

Laboratory Findings: Serum human chorionic gonadotropin positive, fasting glucose 130 mg/dL, hemoglobin A_{1C} 6.8 mg/dL.

Question: What are the risk factors for gestational diabetes?

Answer: Obesity, maternal age of ≥ 25 years, family history of diabetes, prior macrosomia, history of unexplained fetal death, prior episode of gestational diabetes, and Hispanic or African ethnicity.

Discussion: Of these risk factors, the factor most predictive of gestational diabetes is the history of its occurrence during a previous pregnancy. After having gestational diabetes diagnosed in one pregnancy, the rate of recurrence in subsequent pregnancies has been reported to be 52% to 69%.

Gestational diabetes is defined as glucose intolerance that first is diagnosed during pregnancy. It currently is the most common medical complication of pregnancy. It occurs in approximately 3% to 6% of pregnancies in the United States, but the incidence is higher in certain minority populations. In Native Americans, African Americans, and Latinos, the estimated incidence is 10% to 12%. Gestational hyperglycemia is defined as fasting serum glucose of <105 mg/dL, or a 2-hour postprandial serum glucose of >120 mg/dL.

Pregnancy is a diabetogenic state because of pregnancy-induced hormonal and metabolic changes: Pregnancy-induced increases in estrogen, progesterone, prolactin, cortisol, and human placental lactogen induce insulin resistance. There is an increased insulin demand to maintain euglycemia, but the insulin reserve seems to be blunted in gestational diabetes.

Patients with mild hyperglycemia first can be tried on a diabetic diet and spreading out calories into three meals and three snacks. Limiting carbohydrate intake to 15 to 30 g at breakfast can decrease morning secretion of cortisol, which helps to limit the degree of insulin resistance present the next morning. Increase in daily exercise also is helpful to improve overall insulin sensitivity. Patients should exercise at least 3 to 4 days per week for 15 to 30 minutes, maintaining the heart rate at 70% to 80% of the age-adjusted maximal heart rate (patient's age in years minus 220). Strenuous activity should be avoided.

Schaefer-Graf et al found that the rates of major and minor birth defects and genetic syndromes correlated with degree of hyperglycemia at the time of presentation for prenatal care. This was true for patients with gestational diabetes and type 2 diabetes. The degree of severity of the anomalies also increased with increasing degrees of hyperglycemia. There was no trend as to which particular organ system was involved with varying levels of hyperglycemia, although there was a trend for more than one organ system to be in-volved as glucose levels increased. The most commonly affected organ systems were cardiac, musculoskeletal, and central nervous system. After the first trimester, other investigators found that the greatest risks to the fetus are macrosomia and neonatal hypoglycemia. In mothers who have associated hypertension or renal disease, intrauterine growth retardation is the greatest risk. Overall, 4% to 11% of infants are born with major malformations.

A variety of insulin regimens are available for patients requiring it. If glucose values are above the recommended limits two or more times in a 2-week interval, insulin should be tried. Practitioners can try single-dose NPH, or NPH plus multiple doses of regular insulin. One regimen consists of 4 U of regular insulin before meals that have been associated with hyperglycemia and 4 U of NPH at bedtime if fasting hyperglycemia occurs. If the target value is exceeded for 2 consecutive days, the insulin dose related to that value is increased by 2 U. The practitioner should continue to increase the dose by 2 U the following day if the value still is >30 mg/dL above the target. A study by Javanovic et al showed that the use of insulin lispro was associated with fewer episodes of hypoglycemia than was regular insulin. The **goals of management** are to maintain euglycemia as much as possible and to decrease perinatal morbidity and mortality to that of the general population. Although oral hypoglycemic agents have not been used routinely to date, trials are under way to evaluate their safety and efficacy.

The present patient had three risk factors for gestational diabetes: obesity, positive family history, and a prior diagnosis of gestational diabetes with her last pregnancy. Her fasting glucose of 130 mg/dL was in a range of hyperglycemia that put her fetus at risk for development of a birth defect. Her above-normal hemoglobin A_{1C} implied mild-to-moderate hyperglycemia over several weeks of her first trimester; this too indicated some risk of birth defect. Because the patient failed diet and exercise with her last pregnancy, she was started on a diabetic diet plus half of the insulin regimen she required for the first pregnancy. The insulin was titrated over the following week. She was able to maintain euglycemia but gave birth to an infant with a ventricular septal defect that required repair.

Clinical Pearls

1. The risk of and degree of congenital anomalies occurring in gestational diabetes seem to be related to the degree of hyperglycemia in the first trimester.

2. Significant hyperglycemia is associated with congenital anomalies in multiple organ systems, possibly because of a shared biochemical abnormality.

3. The degree of maternal hyperglycemia seems to influence the number of organ systems involved and the severity of the anomalies.

4. Approximately 10% to 15% of patients with gestational diabetes require insulin therapy.

5. Women with type 1 or 2 diabetes should be counseled to maintain euglycemia as much as possible for 2 to 3 months before pregnancy, then throughout pregnancy.

REFERENCES

1. Ryan EA: Pregnancy in diabetes. Med Clin North Am 82: 823–845, 1998.
2. Javanovic L, Ilic S, Pettitt DJ, et al: Metabolic and immunologic effects of insulin lispro in gestational diabetes. Diabetes Care 22:1422–1427, 1999.
3. Anderson AD, Lichorad A: Update in maternity care: Hypertensive disorders, diabetes mellitus, and anemia. Prim Care 27:185–204, 2000.
4. Schaefer-Graf UM, Buchanan TA, Xiang A, et al: Patterns of congenital anomalies and relationship to initial maternal fasting glucose levels in pregnancies complicated by type II and gestational diabetes. Am J Obstet and Gynecol 182:313–320, 2000.
5. Young C, Kuehl TJ, Sulak PJ, Allen SR: Gestational diabetes screening in subsequent pregnancies of previously healthy patients. Am J Obstet and Gynecol 182:1024–1026, 2000.

PATIENT 34

A 49-year-old man with severe hypertension after surgery for ruptured cerebral aneurysm

A 49-year-old man underwent repair of a ruptured middle cerebral artery aneurysm after presenting to the emergency department with altered consciousness, severe headache, and left arm and leg weakness. CT scan showed a subarachnoid hemorrhage and a moderate parenchymal hemorrhage. During his first postoperative day in the intensive care unit, he develops a systolic blood pressure of 220 mmHg.

Physical Examination: Blood pressure 220/106 mmHg, pulse 92, respirations 14, temperature 98.9°F. General: somnolent, but responds to voice. HEENT: normal. Chest: clear. Cardiac: normal. Neurologic: cranial nerves intact, grade 3+/5 weakness of the left arm, grade 4/5 weakness of the left leg. Deep tendon reflexes 3+ of the left upper extremity. Sensation: decreased on the left arm and leg.

Laboratory Findings: CBC: normal. Serum sodium 131 mEq/dL, potassium 3.8 mEq/dL, chloride 98 mg/dL, bicarbonate 22 mEq/dL, urine sodium 175 mEq/24 h, urine osmolality 205 mEq/dL. ECG: normal sinus rhythm with a prolonged Q-T interval.

Question: What is the blood pressure goal after neurosurgery for subarachnoid hemorrhage?

Answer: Preoperatively, increased blood pressure is treated aggressively to limit any potential for rebleeding. The goal for most patients is to keep the mean arterial pressure in their usual range. If this level is not known, the goal for the mean arterial pressure is < 100 mmHg.

Discussion: To help control blood pressure, patients are kept in a dark, quiet room, lying flat, with limited visitors. Factors that can cause rebleeding are hypertension, seizures, pain, and anxiety or agitation. Patients with a previous diagnosis of hypertension are kept on their usual medications; patients with new hypertension can be given esmolol infusions or labetalol. Blood pressures should be brought into the normal range, but hypotension should be avoided. It is standard therapy also to use nimodipine, a dihydropyridine calcium channel blocker that has been shown to decrease the cerebral arterial vasospasm that often accompanies subarachnoid hemorrhage. Limiting the amount of vasospasm in turn decreases the degree of permanent neurologic deficit. Vasospasm can occur in up to 70% of patients, and can cause symptoms in 20–30% and death in 10–20%.

Postoperatively, volume expansion along with blood pressure control has been shown to improve survival by maintaining cerebral perfusion and limiting vasospasm. Blood pressure can be liberalized postoperatively, and some practitioners allow systolic pressures in the range of **160–180 mmHg**. Nimodipine can be continued for approximately 2 to 3 weeks postoperatively to avoid cerebral vasospasm.

Labetalol and hydralazine are first-line agents for treatment of hypertension because they are titrated easily intravenously and do not worsen intracranial pressure. Blood pressure agents that cause systemic vasodilation also cause cerebral vasodilation, which can cause increased intracranial pressure; these agents should be avoided (i.e., nitroprusside).

Any significant hypoxemia, hypercarbia, or acidosis should be treated vigorously because these conditions can worsen cerebral ischemia and cerebral edema. **Triple H therapy** (hypervolemic, hypertensive, hemodilutional therapy) is used by many practitioners to elevate and maintain cerebral blood flow. Langer et al used isotonic saline intravenously in conjunction with albumin boluses, maintaining central venous pressures between 8 and 12 mmHg. Levy and Giannotta used dobutamine therapy with intravenous fluids in conjunction with Swan-Ganz monitoring to maintain an arterial wedge pressure of approximately 14 mmHg. This pressure enhances cardiac output, with presumed improved perfusion of ischemic cerebral tissue. Other common problems after aneurysmal clipping for subarachnoid hemorrhage include seizure, acute hydrocephalus, rebleeding, and syndrome of inappropriate antidiuretic hormone (SIADH).

Practitioners should be acquainted with the clinical signs and symptoms of a ruptured cerebral aneurysm. The most common presentation is headache. The location may vary depending on the site of the bleeding, but it is often sudden in onset ("thunderclap headache") and often described as the worst headache of the patient's life. Patients also may complain of nausea, vomiting, localized weakness or paresthesia, dysphasia, visual loss, or confusion. Physical examination abnormalities include meningismus, change in reflexes, motor deficits, sensory deficits, cranial nerve palsies, anisocoria, and papilledema. Of patients, 39% may have no localizing signs, especially if the hemorrhage is confined to the subarachnoid space. Significant neurologic lateralizing signs can be due to intracerebral clot, ischemia in the territory of the artery with the aneurysm, or hemorrhage into brain tissue. Coma may be the presenting sign in some patients; death may occur within a few minutes if the hemorrhage is massive.

In the present patient, the aneurysm location was the right middle cerebral artery with rupture partly in the subarachnoid space and partly into the brain tissue. The vessel was clipped successfully, but the patient had permanent postoperative neurologic deficits. His hypertension was treated successfully with labetalol, 20 mg intravenously every 4 hours. His mild SIADH was watched and resolved slowly without specific treatment. His hypertension resolved after 48 hours.

Clinical Pearls

1. Patients with systolic blood pressures >180 mmHg should receive antihypertensive therapy with a medication that does not cause systemic vasodilation.

2. Routine management of postoperative patients after subarachnoid hemorrhage includes nimodipine to prevent cerebral vasospasm, an anticonvulsant to prevent seizures, and corticosteroids to decrease vasospasm from inflammatory mechanisms.

3. Nimodipine may decrease cerebral ischemia by a direct neuronal protective effect and by improving collateral flow.

4. Middle cerebral artery aneurysms are the second most common aneurysm site. Intracerebral bleeding is most common with aneurysms at this location. Middle cerebral artery aneurysms often are accompanied by severe neurologic deficits.

REFERENCES

1. Rudehill A, Olsson GL, Sundqvist K, et al: ECG abnormalities in patients with subarachnoid hemorrhage and intracranial tumours. J Neurol Neurosurg Psychiatry 50:1375, 1987.
2. Weir B, MacDonald L: Cerebral vasospasm. Clin Neurosurg 40:40, 1992.
3. Crowell RM, Gress DR, Ogilvy CS, et al: Principles of management of subarachnoid hemorrhage: General management. In Ratcheson RA, Wirth FP, (eds): Concepts in Neurosurgery: Vol. 6. Ruptured Cerebral Aneurysms: Perioperative Management. Baltimore, Williams & Wilkins, 1994.
4. Levy ML, Giannotta SL: Management of vasospasm: Hemodynamic augmentation. In Ratcheson RA, Wirth FP (eds): Ruptured Cerebral Aneurysms: Perioperative Management. Vol 6: Concepts in Neurosurgery. Baltimore, Williams and Wilkins, 1994, pg 134–135.
5. Langer DJ, Zager EL, Flamm ES. Parasurgical management of aneurysmal subarachnoid hemorrhage. In Cruz J (ed): Neurologic and Neurosurgical Emergencies. Philadelphia, W.B. Saunders, 1998, pp 205–241.

PATIENT 35

A 33-year-old woman with a history of anorexia nervosa

A 33-year-old woman with an 8-year history of anorexia nervosa presents to her primary care physician for evaluation of recent near-syncope and weakness. Her weight has been monitored twice a week for several months and has been stable at 90 lb. She participates in a day-hospitalization program for treatment of anorexia. She appears to the physician to look even more gaunt than usual, yet her weight has remained stable.

Physical Examination: Blood pressure 88/60, pulse 46, temperature 97.0°F. Height: 65.5 inches. Weight: 90 lb. General appearance: Marked temporal wasting. Chest: clear. Extremities: no edema. Acrocyanosis of hands and feet. On moving the patient's gown to look at her musculature, exercising weights were found strapped to the upper thighs. Repeat weight without the exercise equipment: 81 lb.

Laboratory Findings: WBC 3600/µL, Hct 32%, platelets 135,000/µL, sodium 132 mEq/dL, potassium 2.7 mEq/dL, phosphorus 1.6 mg/dL, magnesium 0.8 mEq/dL. ECG: sinus bradycardia.

Question: What is the cause of the patient's symptoms?

Diagnosis: Worsening anorexia nervosa with presyncope resulting from volume depletion, possible arrhythmia, and weakness secondary to hypophosphatemia.

Discussion: Anorexia nervosa is an eating disorder chiefly of young healthy women who starve themselves because of morbid fear of gaining weight. The illness is seen primarily in white women from middle-class and upper-class backgrounds. It occurs only rarely in black women, Asian women, or men. The overall prevalence has been estimated to 0.5 to 1.5 per 100,000, although in adolescent white girls from upper-class backgrounds occurrences of 1 per 100 of the population have been reported. The Table lists the DSM IV criteria for anorexia. There are two subtypes of anorexia nervosa: the binge-purge type and the restrictive type. The restrictive type is more common.

DSM IV* Criteria for Anorexia Nervosa

Refusal to maintain weight within a normal
   range for height and age
Intense fear of weight gain
Severe body image disturbance with undue
   emphasis on body shape
Amenorrhea for 3 consecutive months
Body weight <85% of predicted

*Diagnostic and Statistical Manual of Mental Disorders, 4th ed.

In addition to the medical signs listed in the following Table, other signs and symptoms present in moderate-to-severe cases include constipation, cold intolerance, hypotension, orthostasis, hypothermia, peripheral edema, enlarged parotid glands, undetectable body fat, dry scaly skin, and yellowish skin from carotenemia. Multiple laboratory abnormalities can be seen. On ECG, sinus bradycardia is common, as is low voltage; if severe electrolyte abnormalities are present, ventricular ectopy or Q-T interval prolongation can be seen. On echocardiogram, a decreased muscle mass may be evident and an alteration in chamber sizes and presence of mitral valve prolapse. Bone densitometry may reveal osteopenia or frank osteoporosis; this is thought to develop because of chronically low estrogen levels and elevated cortisol levels.

Hematologic abnormalities include anemia, leukopenia, and thrombocytopenia. These abnormalities almost never are severe enough to require treatment and resolve with weight gain. In addition to constipation, common gastrointestinal problems include delayed gastric emptying and, in binge eaters, gastric dilation (seen in the anorexia subtype of binge-purge). Patients with frequent vomiting can develop parotid gland enlargement. The most notable endocrine abnormalities are reduced secretion of luteinizing hormone, follicle-stimulating hormone, and estradiol. A mildly decreased total thyroxine (T_4) but normal free T_4 usually is present. Thyroid-stimulating hormone usually is normal. Patients also often have a low triiodothyronine (T_3), reflecting a decreased peripheral conversion of T_4 to T_3. This decreased conversion is likely an adaptive response to chronic starvation.

Medical Clues Suggesting Anorexia Nervosa

Distorted attitude toward food and weight that
   overrides hunger
No medical illness that could account for weight
   loss
At least two of the following:
   Amenorrhea
   Lanugo hair
   Bradycardia
   Periods of overactivity
   Episodes of bulimia
   Vomiting (may be self-induced)

Metabolic and renal abnormalities depend on the degree of dietary restriction, whether or not the patient is abusing diuretics or laxatives, and whether the patient has frequent vomiting. Hypokalemia, hypochloremia, and metabolic alkalosis are common. In patients abusing laxatives, metabolic acidosis sometimes is present because of loss of bicarbonate in stool. In some chronic laxative abusers, sodium and water losses cause increased renin secretion and secondary hyperaldosteronism, with an associated metabolic alkalosis.

The treatment goals include restoring and maintaining normal weight and use of cognitive psychotherapy to change the underlying thoughts and behaviors regarding food. A physician should be involved in monitoring the patient's status, particularly with regard to cardiac, metabolic, and gastrointestinal systems. Assistance of a nutritionist also is useful. Patients who have had repeated hospitalizations should be considered for long-term partial hospitalization. A wide variety of psychopharmacologic options have been tried; selective serotonin reuptake inhibitors have been of partial benefit in some patients, as has cyproheptadine, an antihistamine that at high doses has relieved depression and stimulated weight gain.

Physicians caring for anorexic patients should be aware of the criteria for hospitalization: weight <70% to 75% of ideal body weight, serum potassium <3.0 mEq/dL with an abnormal ECG, evidence of dehydration, abnormal vital signs such as hypotension or heart rate <35 beats/min, and cardiac arrhythmias. When hospitalized, the patient may need telemetry, especially in the setting of severe electrolyte disturbances, ventricular ectopy on ECG, or severe bradycardia. Refeeding should begin slowly. Patients should be monitored with daily laboratory tests to evaluate for the development of **refeeding syndrome**. In malnutrition, phosphate depletion at the cellular level causes depletion of compounds such as adenosine triphosphate. In the heart, it leads to a depressed stroke volume (and in starvation, a decrease in ventricular mass). With sudden repletion, the increased intravascular volume can cause congestive heart failure. As cellular function increases because of refeeding, serum phosphate may decrease significantly as a result of intracellular use—this can cause delirium, cardiac arrest, or cardiovascular collapse. Serum phosphate levels should be checked daily in the first few days of refeeding.

Typically, patients hospitalized for refeeding receive diets of 800 to 1000 kcal/d, with increases of 200 to 300 kcal every 3 to 4 days as tolerated.

During initial refeeding, patients may gain weight rapidly because of fluid retention and because the resting metabolic rate is decreased. The metabolic rate increases quickly as the patient gains weight.

The present patient had failed three hospitalizations. She also was becoming more adept at hiding her weight loss. She stated that some of the other patients during her hospitalizations shared tips on how to hide food and how to increase exercise without detection by family or friends. She was hospitalized and placed on telemetry to watch for ventricular ectopy. Her potassium, magnesium, and phosphorus were replaced. She admitted to abuse of laxatives. She was watched closely for refeeding syndrome. Initially, her diet was one can of protein drink three times per day. Her pulse during sleep decreased to 28 beats/min; during the day, it was 44 to 50 beats/min. She had unifocal premature ventricular contractions at a rate of 4/min. The premature ventricular contractions resolved with resolution of her electrolyte abnormalities, as did Q-T interval prolongation. The patient was transferred to an intensive inpatient program in a nearby state and gained 16 lb over a 3-month period. On discharge, she entered a partial hospitalization program, but promptly lost 10 lb. Her long-term prognosis is poor.

Clinical Pearls

1. For critically malnourished patients, the physician must pay particular attention to issues such as metabolic abnormalities, volume depletion and possible arrhythmias, and refeeding syndrome.

2. Frequent monitoring of weight, physical examination, and laboratory parameters performed in conjunction with psychotherapy with an expert in eating disorders can improve outcome.

3. There is new evidence that there may be a genetic predisposition that increases risk for becoming anorexic. Other studies point to overprotective parenting and unresolved grief as risk factors.

REFERENCES

1. Newman MM, Halmi KA: The endocrinology of anorexia nervosa and bulimia nervosa. Endocrinol Metab Clin North Am 17:195–212, 1988.
2. American Psychiatric Association: Diagnostic and Statistic Manual of Mental Disorders, 4th ed. Washington, D.C., American Psychiatric Association, 1994, pp 544–545.
3. Halmi KA: Eating Disorders: Anorexia nervosa, bulimia nervosa, and obesity. In Hales KE, Yudofsky SC, Talbott J (eds): American Psychiatric Association Press Textbook of Psychiatry, 2nd ed. Washington, D.C., American Psychiatric Association Press, 1994, pp 857–875.
4. Wiseman C, Harris WA, Halmi KA: Eating disorders. Med Clin North Am 82:145–159, 1998.
5. Brown JM, Mehler PS, Harris RH: Medical complications occurring in adolescents with anorexia nervosa. West J Med 172:189–193, 2000.
6. Mehler PS: Diagnosis and care of patients with anorexia nervosa in primary care settings. Ann Intern Med 134:1048–1059, 2001.

PATIENT 36

A 68-year-old woman with thrombocytopenia undergoing splenectomy

A 68-year-old woman with idiopathic thrombocytopenic purpura (ITP) requires splenectomy because of failure to respond to medical therapy. Her platelets are in the range of 10,000 to 13,000/μL on prednisone therapy preoperatively.

Physical Examination: Vital signs normal. Chest: clear. Cardiac: normal. Abdomen: spleen palpable 2 cm below the left costal margin.

Laboratory Findings: Blood chemistries: normal. WBC 8700/μL, hematocrit 36%, platelets 11,000/μL.

Question: Does the patient need preoperative platelet transfusion?

Diagnosis: Patient with severe ITP awaiting splenectomy.

Discussion: ITP is the most common hematologic disorder necessitating splenectomy. In ITP, the spleen is the main site of antiplatelet antibody production and antibody-sensitized platelet sequestration and destruction. Often, asymptomatic patients with platelet counts >30,000/μL are observed without therapy. Medical therapy is used for patients with platelet counts <30,000/μL or for patients with bleeding risks (i.e., gastrointestinal disease) whose counts are >30,000/μL. Splenectomy is indicated for patients with refractory symptomatic thrombocytopenia despite medical therapy, patients with relapse after initial response to steroid therapy, patients requiring high doses of medication to achieve remission, and patients who cannot tolerate medication.

During surgery, these patients often can tolerate significant levels of thrombocytopenia without significant blood loss because their platelets have been noted to be hyperfunctional. Nonetheless, for severe thrombocytopenia, many clinicians attempt to improve the preoperative platelet count by using a course of intravenous immunoglobulin, infused a few days preoperatively. **Platelet transfusions are not useful preoperatively** because platelet survival is extremely short. Transfusion is beneficial only in the setting of intraoperative or postoperative hemorrhage. This generally occurs when the platelet count is <50,000 cells/μL.

Patients with severe thrombocytopenia also may benefit from another course of intravenous immunoglobulin or steroids in the immediate postoperative period. Platelet counts usually rebound quickly after splenectomy, however.

Laparoscopic splenectomy, which first was performed successfully in 1991, has become increasingly popular. In experienced hands, the procedure has been found to decrease the length of the surgery, decrease the rate of complications, and decrease length of hospital stay. One review of the literature comparing laparoscopic splenectomy with open splenectomy showed that the main difference between the two is the type of complications. Analysis of >450 cases of laparoscopic procedures revealed only one series with severe complications (pulmonary embolism, portal vein thrombosis, and pancreatic fistula). In one review of a large series of open splenectomy, however, the prevalence of severe complications was higher; postoperative subphrenic abscesses requiring reoperation occurred at a rate of 3% to 5%, rebleeding requiring reexploration occurred in 5% to 7% of cases, and embolism occurred in 2% to 6% of patients. Absolute contraindications to laparoscopic splenectomy include severe cardiopulmonary disease and cirrhosis with portal hypertension.

Thrombocytopenia persists in 13% of patients who undergo splenectomy for ITP. One possible reason for postoperative failure to improve is the presence of accessory spleens. To avoid this possibility, many physicians perform radionuclide scanning with radionuclide-labeled autogenous platelets to look for accessory splenic tissue. If such scanning is done in the postoperative setting and is positive for accessory splenic tissue, reoperation is necessary. Factors that have been found to predict clinical response to splenectomy are listed in the Table.

Factors Predictive of Clinical
Response to Splenectomy

Age <40 years
Prior response to steroid therapy
Good response to preoperative immunoglobulin
Predominant splenic sequestration of platelets
Severity of hemorrhagic tendency

Splenectomy is beneficial in ITP likely because of elimination of a major source of antiplatelet antibody synthesis and elimination of a primary site of platelet destruction. A new therapy may help avoid splenectomy in some patients: Intravenous Rh_0 (D) immune globulin (or anti-D antibodies) induces reversible IgC F_c blockade, sparing platelets from destruction by immune phagocytosis. Patients must be RhD positive, and, since the therapy is associated with hemolysis, they must be able to tolerate a decrease in hematocrit. Intravenous Rh_0 (D) immune globulin undoubtedly will play a growing role in delaying and possibly avoiding splenectomy.

With the loss of the spleen, patients become vulnerable to overwhelming infection with encapsulated organisms—in particular, to pneumococci, meningococci, and *Haemophilus influenzae*. Patients require preoperative vaccination against these agents. If the surgery was done as an emergency, the vaccinations should be given as soon as possible postoperatively.

The present patient received intravenous immunoglobulin over a 3-day period preoperatively. Her platelets increased to 23,000/μL. She underwent splenectomy, requiring 2 U of packed red blood cells and two six-packs of platelet concentrate. Her postoperative platelet count increased to 72,000/μL after the first day and to 153,000/μL by postoperative day 4.

Clinical Pearls

1. Overwhelming postsplenectomy infection refers to overwhelming bacteria with encapsulated organisms (pneumococci, meningococci, and *Haemophilus* organisms) thath can occur in splenectomized patients. Patients must receive preoperative pneumococcal, meningococcal, and *Haemophilus influenzae* B vaccines to help reduce the risk.

2. Occurrence of overwhelming postsplenectomy infection is 1.9% to 4.2% with a mortality rate of 30%.

REFERENCES

1. Julia A, Araguas C, Rossello J, et al: Lack of useful clinical predictors of response to splenectomy in patients with chronic idiopathic thrombocytopenic purpura. Br J Haematol 76:250, 1990.
2. Flowers JL, Lefor AT, Steers J, et al: Laparoscopic splenectomy in patients with hematologic diseases. Ann Surg 224:19–34, 1996.
3. Sandler SG: The spleen and splenectomy in immune (idiopathic) thrombocytopenic purpura. Semin Hematol 37(suppl 1):10–12, 2000.
4. Bennet CL: The potential for treatment of idiopathic thrombocytopenia purpura with anti-D to prevent splenectomy: A predictive cost analysis. Semin Hematol 37(suppl 1):26–30, 2000.
5. Katkhouda N, Mavor E: Laparoscopic splenectomy. Surg Clin North Am 80:1285–1298, 2000.

PATIENT 37

A 61-year-old man with recent coronary artery stenting, now requiring noncardiac surgery

A 61-year-old man underwent percutaneous transluminal coronary artery angioplasty and stent implantation of a 90% left anterior stenosis. At that time, he had presented with substernal chest pain with radiation to the jaw. His peak creatine phosphokinase was 608 mg/dL with a troponin I of 3.7 ng/mL. He did well on the postinfarction exercise treadmill test and was sent home on aspirin, atorvastatin (Lipitor), metoprolol, and clopidogrel. Twelve days later, he underwent emergent left colectomy for severe diverticular bleeding. During colectomy, bleeding was moderate because the patient had been on two antiplatelet agents (aspirin and clopidogrel). He required transfusion of a six-pack of platelets and 2 U of packed red blood cells. Aspirin and clopidogrel had been held for 24 hours preoperatively and were held for 24 hours postoperatively. Early on the second postoperative day, the patient develops substernal chest pain radiating to the jaw, hypotension, and tachycardia. The ECG reveals 3-mm ST segment elevation in leads V1 through V4.

Physical Examination: Blood pressure 82/50, pulse 122. General appearance: diaphoretic and pale. Jugular venous distention: 3 cm. Chest: bibasilar rales. Heart: tachycardic. No murmurs or gallops. Abdomen: hypoactive bowel sounds. Tender at the surgical site. Surgical wound clean and dry.

Laboratory Findings: ECG: tachycardia with 3-mm ST elevation of V1 through V4. 2-mm ST depression of leads I, aVL, V5, and V6. Electrolytes: sodium 134 mEq/dL, potassium 3.5 mEq/dL, bicarbonate 26 mEq/dL. BUN 28 mg/dL, creatinine 1.5 mg/dL. Creatine phosphokinase 600 mg/dL, MB fraction pending, troponin 6.9 ng/dL.

Question: What are the recommendations for proceeding with noncardiac surgery after coronary stenting?

Answer: Because of the risk of coronary thrombosis at the site of the stent, the current recommendations are to wait 4 weeks after stenting unless the surgery is urgent.

Discussion: Studies have shown that noncardiac surgery performed within 2 weeks of coronary artery stenting is associated with a high risk of stent thrombosis, with subsequent myocardial infarction and risk of death. Kaluza et al reported a series of 40 patients who underwent major noncardiac surgery shortly after percutaneous transluminal coronary angioplasty (PTCA) with coronary stent implantation. Of 40 patients, 25 had surgery <2 weeks after stenting, and 15 had surgery between 2 and 6 weeks after stenting. All patients had aspirin and ticlopidine continued after stenting. Almost all patients had their anticoagulants held for 0 to 24 hours preoperatively and 0 to 24 hours postoperatively. Seven patients experienced postoperative myocardial infarctions, and of these, six died. Eleven patients experienced major bleeding, and two patients died as a result of complications related to the bleeding.

Major surgery is known to induce a hypercoagulable state, and coronary artery stents are known to be thrombogenic. (In fact, one of the patients who suffered postoperative cardiac death in the Kaluza series was kept on his antithrombogenic regimen throughout the perioperative period). It has been postulated that the abrupt withdrawal of poststenting antithrombotic medication may contribute to the high rate of acute intrastent thrombosis. Based on the current information, it is wise to delay surgery whenever possible until 2 to 4 weeks after coronary artery stenting, when the poststenting antithrombotic regimen is completed. Even so, Vicenzi et al reported an episode of infarction 32 days after stent implantation.

The implications of these reports complicates the task of preoperative cardiac risk assessment. Past studies have shown a reduction of perioperative cardiac complications and postoperative cardiac death with coronary artery bypass graft surgery and PTCA. Similar perioperative reduction of risk does not seem to be conferred by preoperative PTCA with stent implantation. This finding may have a great impact on perioperative cardiac management and timing of surgery because stents now are used so frequently (>50% of all PTCA procedures). Because PTCA alone, without stenting, has been reported to result in fewer perioperative cardiac complications and has not been associated with the same risk of catastrophic thrombosis on cessation of antiplatelet therapy, patients undergoing preoperative cardiac PTCA probably should not have stents implanted if surgery must take place within 2 to 4 weeks after PTCA.

The present patient experienced an acute myocardial infarction postoperatively. He underwent immediate cardiac catheterization, when he was found to have complete stent thrombosis. He underwent redilation successfully to a 30% stenosis.

Clinical Pearls

1. Coronary artery stenting seems to create a high degree of perioperative cardiac risk if subsequent surgery is done before poststenting antithrombotic therapy is completed.

2. When major noncardiac surgery is performed during the period of antithrombotic therapy, the patient also is at risk for major bleeding.

3. When subsequent surgery is performed several months after PTCA (without stenting), the rates of myocardial infarction and death are comparable to results achieved with coronary artery bypass graft surgery.

REFERENCES
1. Huber KC, Evans MA, Breshanan JF, et al: Outcome of noncardiac operations in patients with severe coronary artery disease successfully treated preoperatively with coronary angioplasty. Mayo Clin Proc 67:15–21, 1992.
2. Elmore JR, Halett Jr JW, Gibbons RJ, et al: Myocardial revascularization before abdominal aortic aneurysmorrhaphy: Effect of coronary angioplasty. Mayo Clin Proc 68:637–641, 1993.
3. Kaluza GL, Joseph J, Lee JR, et al: Catastrophic outcomes of noncardiac surgery soon after coronary stenting. J Am Coll Cardiol 35:1288–1294, 2000.
4. Hassan SA, Hlatky MA, Boothroyd DB, et al: Outcomes of noncardiac surgery after coronary bypass surgery or coronary angioplasty in the Bypass Angioplasty Revascularization Investigation (BARI). Am J Med 110:260–266, 2001.
5. Vicenzi MN, Ribitsch D, Luha O, et al: coronary artery stenting before noncardiac surgery: More threat than safety? Anesthesiology 94:367–368, 2001.

PATIENT 38

A 76-year-old woman with Parkinson's disease undergoing repair of a fractured hip

A 76-year-old woman with Parkinson's disease underwent pinning the right hip after sustaining a hip fracture in a fall. She has moderately persistent parkinsonian symptoms with her current medication regimen. Six hours after surgery, she is not taking anything orally because of nausea, vomiting, and confusion. She is noted to have worsening stiffness and bilateral upper extremity tremor. The tremor is causing enough movement of the rest of her body that it is worsening her pain at the surgical site.

Physical Examination: Temperature 99.2°F, pulse 88, respirations 12, blood pressure 108/62. General appearance: Confused to place and time. Chest: clear. Cardiac: normal. Neurologic: masked facies. Extremities moderately stiff. 2+ cogwheeling at the wrists. Bilateral upper extremity resting tremors. Unable to test gait. No motor or sensory deficits.

Laboratory Findings: Electrolytes and CBC normal. BUN 22 mg/dL, creatine 1.3 mg/dL. Oxygen saturation 90% at room air.

Question: What postoperative problems do patients with Parkinson's disease face?

Answer: Postoperatively, these patients are at risk for aspiration pneumonia, respiratory muscle insufficiency, delirium, and worsening of parkinsonian symptoms.

Discussion: One of the major problems for patients with Parkinson's disease in the postoperative setting is that the most effective medications for the disease are **oral formulations,** with no intravenous or intramuscular forms available. Significant worsening of symptoms can occur when patients are NPO (taking nothing by mouth) after surgery.

A rebounding of parkinsonian symptoms can occur after missing only one dose, and untreated patients also can develop a **dopamine withdrawal syndrome,** which resembles neuroleptic malignant syndrome. This syndrome generally occurs 24 to 72 hours after abrupt cessation of a dopamine agent and is thought to be caused by acute cerebral dopamine depletion. The major symptoms are fever, muscular rigidity, delirium or coma, and autonomic instability. The mainstay of treatment is to restart dopaminergic medications. Patients more commonly manifest a worsening of parkinsonian symptoms because their oral medications are being held while they are NPO, but they generally do not develop a full withdrawal syndrome.

All of the major antiparkinsonian medications are in the oral form, making perioperative NPO patients difficult to treat. On resuming oral intake, patients with Parkinson's disease often have a period of decreased responsiveness to treatment postoperatively. This phenomenon is not well understood and may be due in part to a residual effect of anesthetics and analgesics and slowed gastric emptying with a subsequent decreased delivery of levodopa.

Patients also have an increased risk of **aspiration** postoperatively. These patients already tend to have sialorrhea and pharyngeal muscle dysfunction. Postoperatively, in the face of sedation and lack of usual medication, pooling of saliva in the posterior pharynx and swallowing dysfunction can increase, leading to an increased risk of aspiration. Routine aspiration precautions should be undertaken. Some patients with **Parkinson's disease** have mild restrictive pulmonary defects because of stiffness of the chest wall musculature. This stiffness can worsen postoperatively and lead to **hypoxemia.** Oxygen saturation values should be followed, and supplemental oxygen should be given as needed.

A significant problem for some patients is the development of **postoperative delirium and psychosis.** Patients most at risk are those with Parkinson's-associated dementia. The delirium can be associated with alterations in the usual regimen of antiparkinsonian medications, metabolic abnormalities, or use of a provocative medication such has an anticholinergic. In addition, the use of various anesthetics and analgesics with antiparkinsonian drugs may induce delirium. Haloperidol and fluphenazine may worsen parkinsonian symptoms and should be avoided if possible. If an antipsychotic is necessary, mesoridazine or thioridazine can be tried. For hallucinations in these patients, ondansetron has been reported to be useful.

For patients who are nauseous, nasogastric suctioning alone may be sufficient. If additional therapy is necessary, ondesetron or domperidone can be tried. For patients who are NPO but have significant tremor, trihexyphenidyl, starting at 0.5 to 1.0 mg intravenously twice a day, is an option, given with benztropine twice a day to limit side effects. For patients with dementia, however, cognitive status may worsen because of the anticholinergic properties of these medications. For rigidity, amantadine, 100 mg twice a day, can be helpful.

For patients who have significant alteration of consciousness, dysphagia, or abnormality of the upper gastrointestinal tract, their usual oral medications can be delivered through a weighted Silastic feeding tube so that medications may be delivered to the duodenum. If there is long-term inability to take oral medication in a patient with severe disease, use of a percutaneous jejunostomy feeding tube can be considered. Levodopa and carbidopa solution can be prepared by pulverizing and dissolving 4 tablets of regular carbidopa/levodopa (25/250 strength) in 1000 mL of water with 1000 mg of vitamin C to produce a 1 mg/mL solution of levodopa. The infusion can start at 25 mL/h (i.e., for a patient on levodopa, 100 mg every 4 hours), then titrated. Higher starting doses are required for patients using higher amounts of preoperative levodopa. A dark bottle should be used to protect the solution from light, and it should be refrigerated. The solution is stable for at least 24 hours.

The present patient was given ondansetron so that she could tolerate her oral medications more quickly. She also was given trihexyphenidyl and benztropine to help her tremor. These agents seemed to worsen her postoperative confusion, but gave her some relief from the tremor and relief from tremor-related pain at the operative site. Amantadine was added to help limit her stiffness in an effort to reduce associated postoperative hypoxia. She was given supplemental oxygen, which improved her oxygen saturation to 94%. She was able to take her usual oral medications after 24 hours, with subsequent improved control of parkinsonian symptoms. Her postoperative confusion lasted 7 days. She received thioridazine with some benefit.

Clinical Pearls

1. Patients with Parkinson's disease should have resumption of oral medications as soon as possible after surgery.

2. Sudden and prolonged withdrawal of levodopa can cause a dopamine withdrawal syndrome, which clinically resembles neuroleptic malignant syndrome. Bromocriptine, diazepam, and dantrolene are treatment options and reinstitution of levodopa as soon as possible.

3. Oxygen saturation should be monitored closely in these patients to evaluate for postoperative hypoventilation from respiratory muscle rigidity.

4. Patients who use selegiline (Eldepryl) for Parkinson's disease should not receive meperidine (Demerol) perioperatively. The combination of these medications can cause delirium and can cause symptoms similar to neuroleptic malignant syndrome. Some anesthesiologists recommend stopping selegiline a few days before surgery to avoid potential drug interactions.

REFERENCES

1. Kurlan R, Nutt JG, Woodward WR, et al: Duodenal and gastric delivery of levodopa in parkinsonism. Ann Neurol 22:589–595, 1988.
2. Golden WE, Lavender RC, Metzer WS: Acute postoperative confusion and hallucinations in Parkinson disease. Ann Intern Med 3:218–222, 1989.
3. Reed AP, Han DG: Intraoperative exacerbation of Parkinson's disease. Anesth Analg 75:850–853, 1992.
4. Scuderi P, Wetchler B, Sung Y-F, et al: Treatment of postoperative nausea and vomiting after outpatient surgery with the 5-Ht3 antagonist ondansetron. Anesthesiology 78:15–20, 1993.
5. Juncos JL: Parkinson's disease. In Lubin MF, Walker HK, Smith III RB (eds): Medical Management of the Surgical Patient, 3rd ed. Philadelphia, J.B. Lippincott, 1995, pp 388–396.

PATIENT 39

A 67-year-old diabetic man with respiratory arrest after elective surgery

A 67-year-old diabetic man underwent an elective total hip replacement without intraoperative complication. One hour after surgery, the patient becomes hypotensive (blood pressure 66/42 mmHg) and bradycardic (pulse 52 beats/min). The ECG does not reveal any ischemic changes. He becomes suddenly apneic, requiring reintubation. His medical history is notable for type 2 diabetes mellitus for the past 25 years, peripheral neuropathy secondary to diabetes, and hypertension. He has no history of lung disease and has never smoked. Before surgery, he had no respiratory complaints.

Physical Examination: Temperature 98.9°F, pulse 78, respirations 16, blood pressure 128/70. General appearance: sedated but responsive. Chest: clear. Cardiac: normal. Abdomen: soft, nontender, no masses.

Laboratory Findings (after intubation): ABG: pH 7.43, $PaCO_2$ 38 mmHg, PaO_2 253 mmHg. Chest radiograph: no abnormalities. ECG: no ischemic changes. Head CT scan: normal. Blood chemistries: normal. Glucose: 205 mg/dL, D-dimer <500.

Questions: What was the cause of the patient's respiratory arrest? Is this type of reaction preventable?

Diagnosis: Autonomic neuropathy with postoperative respiratory arrest in a diabetic patient.

Discussion: Autonomic neuropathy has been a reported finding in 20% to 40% of all diabetics. The finding of autonomic neuropathy puts patients at risk for sudden perioperative bradycardia, hypotension, cardiac arrest, and respiratory arrest. Ewing et al[1] reported significantly greater morbidity and mortality in a group of diabetics with autonomic neuropathy compared with patients with diabetes of equal severity and duration who had normal autonomic function.

Cardiorespiratory arrest in diabetics with autonomic dysfunction has occurred spontaneously and in the perioperative setting. Page and Watkins[2] reported on 12 episodes of cardiorespiratory arrest in eight hospitalized patients. Three of the episodes occurred during anesthesia, and two occurred in the recovery room. In all but one case, there was rapid response to cardiopulmonary resuscitation. All of the episodes occurred in the absence of cardiac dysrhythmia or infarction.

There have been reports of abnormalities in cardiovascular innervation and respiratory reflexes in diabetics. Also, in familial dysautonomia, it has been shown that ventilatory responses to hypoxia and hypercapnia are impaired: Hypoxia can cause syncope, bradycardia, hypotension, and seizures, whereas a sudden increase in oxygen concentration for treatment of hypoxia can induce apnea.

Similarly, ventilatory reflexes in diabetic patients with autonomic neuropathy often are abnormal. Affected diabetics likely have decreased respiratory response to hypoxia and may be particularly sensitive to drugs with respiratory depressant effects. Also, high concentrations of oxygen may induce periods of apnea in these patients.

In the perioperative setting, the cardiopulmonary arrests that occurred in these patients all have been either intraoperative or in the immediate postoperative period. **There is no treatment to prevent these episodes;** watchful waiting and intensive monitoring are paramount. Patients should remain in the recovery room postoperatively for at least 3 hours.

In diabetics, preoperative evaluation should include evaluation for peripheral neuropathy because patients with autonomic insufficiency almost always have coexistent peripheral neuropathy if autonomic testing cannot be done easily. Office-based autonomic tests include the cold pressor test (evaluation for increased blood pressure and heart rate after the patient's hand is in an ice water bath for 60 seconds) and evaluating respiratory sinus arrhythmia on an ECG. Patients with normal autonomic function have a variation in heart rate of at least 15 beats/min when comparing the heart rate between maximal inspiration and maximal expiration. Patients with autonomic insufficiency lose this response and have a respiratory sinus arrhythmia (beat-to-beat variability) of ≤ 5. To test this, a continuous ECG rhythm strip is performed. During a 1-minute interval, the patient should perform a period of forceful breathing at a frequency of 6 breaths/min. The clinician marks on the ECG rhythm strip the R-R interval at which maximal expiration and maximal inspiration occur. Over the 1-minute period, there are six cycles, which can be averaged. Divide 60 by the R-R interval in milliseconds; this gives the heart rate at that moment. The difference between the heart rate at maximal inspiration and maximal expiration should be at least 15, although, it may be slightly lower in elderly patients. If it is ≤ 5, significant autonomic insufficiency is present.

In the present patient, after treatment with ephedrine and then phenylephrine (Neo-Synephrine), the blood pressure and pulse improved to 128/70 mmHg and 78 beats/min. The patient extubated himself 90 minutes after his respiratory arrest and had normal respirations. The rest of his hospital course was uneventful. Performance of a rhythm strip with forceful breathing done later as an outpatient showed a respiratory sinus arrhythmia of only 2 beats/min.

Clinical Pearls

1. Patients with long-standing diabetes mellitus, especially if they have diabetic neuropathy, may have coexisting autonomic neuropathy and are at risk for sudden perioperative cardiac or pulmonary arrest. The anesthesiologist should be notified of this possibility.

2. Preoperative evaluation for autonomic neuropathy can include cold pressor test, evaluation for postural orthostasis, blood pressure response to the Valsalva maneuver, and evaluation of respiratory sinus variation on rhythm strip.

3. If specific autonomic testing cannot be done in the office, the patient should be tested for signs and symptoms of peripheral neuropathy, and the review of the systems should be evaluated for autonomic neuropathy (presence of impotence, dysphagia, delayed gastric emptying, diarrhea [especially nocturnal], orthostasis, and syncope). If autonomic neuropathy is suspected, the anesthesiologist should be notified.

REFERENCES

1. Ewing DJ, Campbell IW, Clarke BF: Mortality in diabetic autonomic neuropathy. Lancet 1:601–603, 1976.
2. Page M McB, Watkins PJ: Cardiorespiratory arrest and diabetic autonomic neuropathy. Lancet 1:14–16, 1978.
3. Burgos LG, Ebert TJ, Asiddao C, et al: Increased intraoperative cardiovascular morbidity in diabetics with autonomic neuropathy. Anesthesiology 70:591–597, 1989.
4. Charlson ME, MacKenzie R, Gold JP: Preoperative autonomic function abnormalities in patients with diabetes mellitus and patients with hypertension. J Am Coll Surg 179:1–10, 1994.

PATIENT 40

A 25-year-old pregnant woman with an acute asthmatic exacerbation

A 25-year-old pregnant woman at 12 weeks' gestation with a 10-year history of intermittent severe asthma presents with a 48-hour history of increased dyspnea, wheezing, and cough. She denies fever, sputum, or chest pain, and there is no personal or family history suggestive of a thrombophilia. Her asthma has been controlled easily in the past by use of inhaled beclomethasone, 2 puffs four times a day, and salmeterol, 2 puffs twice a day. She stopped both of these medications when she first found out she was pregnant and has been taking her albuterol inhaler only when she felt she "absolutely had to."

Physical Examination: Temperature 37°C, pulse 120, respirations 34, blood pressure 110/65. General appearance: In mild distress but able to speak in full sentences. Skin: no lesions. HEENT: normal. Chest: rapid labored breathing but no intercostal indrawing or accessory muscle use seen. Diffuse wheezing heard on auscultation of the chest but no crackles or rubs heard. Cardiac: regular tachycardia with normal heart sounds, but a nonradiating grade III/VI ejection systolic murmur is heard at the left upper sternal border. Abdomen: normal. Extremities: no edema. Neuromuscular: normal.

Laboratory Findings: CBC: WBC 12,000/μL with a normal differential, hemoglobin 11.0 g/dL, platelets 185,000/μL. Blood chemistries normal. ECG: sinus tachycardia, otherwise normal. ABG (room air): pH 7.34, $PaCO_2$ 30 mmHg, PaO_2 96 mmHg. Peak flow is measured at 200.

Questions: How should you manage this patient's asthma in view of the fact that she is pregnant? What is your interpretation of the blood gas values?

Answer: Asthma management is largely unchanged by pregnancy. The patient's blood gas values are normal; in pregnancy normal PaO_2 = 90–100 mmHg, and normal $PaCO_2$ = 28–32 mmHg.

Discussion: Pregnant patients with asthma can expect good pregnancy outcomes if their asthma is well controlled. Poorly controlled asthma can result in an increased risk of perinatal complications. Active treatment of asthma in pregnancy is to be encouraged. If indicated, a chest radiograph can be done safely throughout pregnancy, although in this case one does not seem to be necessary to the diagnosis.

Most available data suggest the usual agents used to treat asthma in pregnancy seem to be well tolerated by the human embryo and fetus (see Table). The only commonly used asthma agents that should *not* be routinely employed in pregnancy are the leukotriene inhibitors (e.g., montelukast, zafirlukast, and particularly zileuton), unless these agents have been essential to control of the patient's asthma in the past. Inhaled bronchodilators, inhaled and systemic steroids, theophylline preparations, ipratropium, and cromolyn all can be used comfortably in the pregnant patient. Among the inhaled corticosteroids, beclomethasone is the preferred agent, but more potent inhaled steroids may be used when clinically necessary for asthma control. Theophylline preparations routinely need dose adjustments in pregnancy because of altered pharmacokinetics. Use of epinephrine should be *avoided* except in a true emergency, because epinephrine-related vasoconstriction can cause acute decreases in placental blood flow.

The present patient was placed on oxygen to maintain an oxygen saturation of $\geq$ 95% and was given three back-to-back treatments of albuterol followed by a treatment with inhaled ipratropium. Her peak flows improved to 250. She subsequently was given methylprednisolone, 125 mg intravenously every 8 hours and admitted to the hospital. Two days later, she was much improved and was sent home on a tapering course of prednisone and her previous regimen of daily inhaled beclomethasone and salmeterol.

Pregnancy Safety Data About the Most Commonly Used Asthma Medications

Class	Agent	Effect on Embryo and Fetus
Short-acting inhaled β_2-adrenergic agonists	Albuterol Isoproterenol Metaproterenol Terbutaline	Published experience with these drugs in humans suggests that β-sympathomimetics do not increase the risk of congenital anomalies. Albuterol is the most studied of these agents. Metaproterenol is the second most studied and terbutaline is the least studied
Long-acting inhaled β-adrenergic agonists	Salmeterol	Animal data of intravenously administered salmeterol have not been reassuring, but this agent is thought probably to be safe in humans when administered by inhalation. No human data about this agent have been published at this point, however, and the use of this agent should be reserved for patients who have failed low-potency steroids or cromolyn alone
Inhaled anticholinergic	Ipratropium	Reassuring animal studies exist, but no published human data. Efficacy in acute asthma attacks, presenting to the emergency department makes its short-term use seem justifiable
Inhaled corticosteroids	Low potency: beclomethasone Medium potency: trimacinolone High potency: fluticasone, budenoside	Beclomethasone is the most widely studied of the inhaled corticosteroids in pregnancy and should be considered the preferred inhaled steroid in pregnancy. Having a nearly identical structure to betamethasone, beclomethasone does cross the placenta. Human data have not suggested any teratogenic effects of this agent Triamcinolone is the next most studied inhaled steroid in pregnancy with this limited experience suggesting no adverse pregnancy effects

116

Class	Agent	Effect on Embryo and Fetus
		Safety data on budenoside are limited, but use for severe asthma not responsive to lower potency steroids seems justifiable given limited systemic absorption
		Fluticasone has not been studied in pregnancy, but use when indicated is generally clinically justifiable.
Mast cell stabilizers	Cromolyn sodium Nedocromil	Human and animal data suggest these agents are not teratogens. Cromolyn has been evaluated better in human pregnancy than nedocromil and should be considered the preferred agent of this class
Leukotriene antagonists	Zileuton Zafirlukast Montelukast	The leukotriene antagonists represent an exception to the general rule that asthma treatment is largely unchanged in pregnancy. Zafirlukast and montelukast have favorable animal data, but data about their safety in human pregnancy are extremely limited at this point. Zileuton has concerning animal data associated with it. Their use should be limited in pregnancy to unusual cases in which a woman has had significant improvement in asthma control with these medications before becoming pregnant that was not obtainable through other methods
Theophyllines	Theophylline Aminophylline	Theophylline and its intravenous form aminophylline do not seem to be human teratogens. Altered pharmacokinetics in pregnancy make monitoring of serum levels and dose adjustments essential
Systemic steroids	Oral: prednisone Intravenous: methyl-prednisolone, hydrocortisone	Most data suggest that systemic steroids do not present a teratogenic risk in pregnancy. A case-control study found, however, a significant association with first-trimester use and oral clefts (odds ratio = 6.55, 95% confidence interval = 1.44–29.76). Even if this association is real, the benefits of controlling a life-threatening disease makes steroid use when indicated in the first trimester still generally justifiable

Clinical Pearls

1. Active treatment of asthma in pregnancy is important to ensure a good outcome for the mother and fetus.

2. The use of inhaled β-agonists, inhaled steroids, systemic steroids, theophyllines, inhaled ipratropium, and inhaled cromolyn is justifiable to treat asthma in pregnancy. Leukotriene antagonists should be avoided during pregnancy at this time unless their perceived benefit for a particular patient outweighs the paucity of human pregnancy data for these agents.

REFERENCES

1. Dombrowski MP: Pharmacologic therapy of asthma during pregnancy. Obstet Gynecol Clin North Am 24:559–574, 1997.
2. Schatz M, Zeiger RS, Harden K, et al: The safety of asthma and allergy medications during pregnancy. J Allergy Clin Immunol 100:301–306, 1997.
3. Rodriguez-Pinilla E, Martinez-Frias ML: Corticosteroids during pregnancy and oral clefts: A case-control study. Teratology 58:2–5, 1998.
4. Luskin AT: An overview of the recommendations of the Working Group on Asthma and Pregnancy. National Asthma Education and Prevention Program. J Allergy Clin Immunol 103(pt 2):S350–353, 1999.
5. Schatz M: Asthma and pregnancy. Lancet 353:1202–1204, 1999.
6. American College of Obstetricians and Gynecologists (ACOG) and American College of Allergy, Asthma and Immunology (ACAAI): The use of newer asthma and allergy medications during pregnancy. Ann Allergy Asthma Immunol 84:475–480, 2000.

PATIENT 41

A 38-year-old pregnant woman with unexplained sudden onset of dyspnea and chest pain

A 38-year-old gravida 3, para 0 pregnant woman at 24 weeks' gestation who has had no previous significant medical history presents with sudden onset of dyspnea and right-sided pleuritic chest pain occurring after a plane trip home from a visit to her relatives in Bucharest. She denies fever, chills, or chest pain. There is no family history suggestive of a thrombophilia, but she did lose both prior pregnancies to late first-trimester miscarriages.

Physical Examination: Temperature 98.6°F, pulse 104, respirations 22, blood pressure 105/70. Patients appears to be in only mild distress. Skin: no lesions. HEENT: normal. Chest: no chest wall tenderness. Mild tachypnea but otherwise completely normal examination. No crackles or rubs heard. Cardiac: regular minimal tachycardia with normal heart sounds, but a nonradiating grade III/VI ejection systolic murmur is heard at the left upper sternal border. Abdomen: normal. Extremities: no edema. Neuromuscular: normal.

Laboratory Findings: CBC: WBC 8000/μL with a normal differential, hemoglobin 10.8 mmol/L, platelets 167,000/μL. Blood chemistries:normal. ECG: sinus tachycardia; otherwise normal. ABG (room air): pH 7.34, $PaCO_2$ 28 mmHg (normal in pregnancy is 28 to 32 mmHg), PaO_2 90 mmHg (normal in pregnancy at sea level is 90 to 100 mmHg). Arterial-alveolar gradient 25 mmHg. Chest radiograph: normal.

Questions: How should this patient be investigated further? What is the relevance of her obstetric history? What is the most likely diagnosis, and how would you manage that possibility in pregnancy?

Diagnosis and Treatment: Probable acute pulmonary embolism despite unremarkable physical and laboratory examination. Further evaluation with a ventilation-perfusion scan followed by angiogram for equivocal cases should occur. If pulmonary embolism is identified, treatment with intravenous heparin acutely followed by twice-daily injections of either unfractionated or low-molecular-weight heparin for the duration of pregnancy is advisable. Warfarin should not be used.

Discussion: Thromboembolism is one of the leading causes of maternal mortality in the Western world. The risk of thromboembolic disease is increased 3-fold to 7-fold throughout gestation and for 6 weeks postpartum.

The presentation of pulmonary embolism in pregnancy often is more subtle than among nonpregnant patients with comorbid medical conditions. Arterial blood gases in particular may be normal (see normal values for pregnancy under Laboratory Findings). A high index of suspicion must be maintained for thromboembolic disease in pregnancy. A particularly high index of suspicion should exist when there is a family history of thromboembolic disease. A family history of thrombosis suggests the possibility an inherited thrombophilia (i.e., deficiency of protein S, protein C, or antithrombin 3; mutations in the genes for prothrombin, factor V, or methylenetetrahydrofolate reductase). Similarly a history of adverse obstetric outcomes, such as preeclampsia occurring at <34 weeks' gestation, recurrent miscarriages, or intrauterine growth restriction, is suggestive of an inherited thrombotic tendency or an acquired one, such as antiphospholipid antibodies or the lupus anticoagulant.

Investigation for pulmonary embolism or deep venous thrombosis in pregnancy should be the same as if the patient were not pregnant. Radiation exposure from chest radiographs, ventilation-perfusion scans, angiogram, and spiral CT scan is well below acceptable standards of safety. Even if all these tests are done, the cumulative radiation dose is well within accepted standards. Appropriate investigation of pulmonary embolism should not be withheld because of concerns about fetal effects of testing.

If pulmonary embolism or deep venous thrombosis is diagnosed during pregnancy, treatment should be with either unfractionated or low-molecular-weight heparin. If unfractionated heparin is used, the patient is given twice-daily (every 12 hours) injections of heparin with a goal of achieving an activated partial thromboplastin time of 60 to 80 seconds midway (6 hours) between the doses. If low-molecular-weight heparin is used, dosing can be based on weight, but many investigators suggest that midinterval heparin levels still should be checked because heparin pharmacokinetics may be altered in pregnancy. The platelet count should be followed with initial heparin therapy because of the risk of heparin-induced thrombocytopenia. Prolonged use of heparin in pregnancy has been associated with a reversible loss in bone density, which in rare cases has caused osteoporotic fractures. Heparin-induced thrombocytopenia and bone density loss may be less common with low-molecular-weight heparin. Warfarin cannot be used because it is a known teratogen in the first trimester and is associated with cerebral malformations if used in the last two trimesters. Warfarin is, however, compatible with breast-feeding. Duration of treatment is 6 months, but because the risk of recurrence remains high until 6 weeks postpartum, continuation of anticoagulation until 6 weeks postpartum is encouraged.

The present patient had a ventilation-perfusion scan, which was read as high probability for pulmonary embolism. She was treated initially with intravenous heparin, then switched to heparin, 12,000 U subcutaneously every 12 hours, which achieved a therapeutic midinterval activated partial thromboplastin time of 65 seconds. Heparin was held when the patient went into labor 16 weeks later at 40 weeks' gestation. She had a normal spontaneous delivery of a healthy 7-lb girl. Postpartum, the patient was switched over to warfarin, which she stayed on for the final 8 weeks of her therapy. Despite her pulmonary embolism and two previous miscarriages, no thrombophilia was identified on subsequent testing.

Clinical Pearls

1. Pregnancy is a risk factor for thromboembolic disease.
2. A high index of suspicion for thromboembolic disease in pregnancy must be maintained because its presentation may be subtler than that seen in the general medical population.
3. Investigation of thromboembolic disease is unchanged in pregnancy and can be carried out with confidence that the levels of radiation used should not harm the fetus.
4. Warfarin should not be used in pregnancy; acute thromboembolic disease in pregnancy should be treated with heparin.

REFERENCES

1. Casele HL, Laifer SA, Woelkers DA, Venkataramanan R: Changes in the pharmacokinetics of the low-molecular-weight heparin enoxaparin sodium during pregnancy. Am J Obstet Gynecol 181(pt 1):1113–1117, 1999.
2. Kupferminc MJ, Eldor A, Steinman N, et al: Increased frequency of genetic thrombophilia in women with complications of pregnancy. N Engl J Med 340:9–13, 1999.
3. Sanson BJ, Lensing AW, Prins MH, et al: Safety of low-molecular-weight heparin in pregnancy: A systematic review. Thromb Haemost 81:668–672, 1999.
4. Chan WS, Chunilal SD, Ginsberg AS: Antithrombotic therapy during pregnancy. Semin Perinatol 25:165–169, 2001.
5. Ginsberg JS, Greer I, Hirsh J: Use of antithrombotic agents during pregnancy. Chest 119(suppl):122S–131S, 2001.

PATIENT 42

A 32-year-old pregnant woman with hypertension presenting at 33 weeks' gestation

A 32-year-old gravida 1, para 0 pregnant woman who has had no previous significant medical history is noted to have a blood pressure of 155/90 mmHg at her prenatal visit at 33 weeks' gestation. Her blood pressures were not noted to be elevated earlier in the pregnancy. She had only limited episodic medical care prior to being pregnant, and does not know what her pre-pregnancy blood pressures were. She reports no headache, visual symptoms, or epigastric pain.

Physical Examination: Temperature 98.6°F, pulse 88, respirations 12, blood pressure now 160/90. Patient appears comfortable. Skin: no lesions. HEENT: no retinal vasospasm or edema on funduscopic examination. Chest: completely clear to auscultation and percussion. Cardiac: regular pulse with normal heart sounds Abdomen: normal. Extremities: mild bilateral peripheral lower limb edema. Neuromuscular: reflexes brisk but no clonus demonstrated.

Laboratory Findings: CBC: normal. Electrolytes: normal. Creatinine 0.8 mg/dL, uric acid 4.3 mg/dL, aspartate aminotransferase (AST) 34 U/L. Urinalysis: 1+ proteinuria. ECG: normal.

Questions: What is the differential diagnosis? How would you manage this woman's blood pressure while she is pregnant?

Diagnosis and Treatment: Pregnancy-induced hypertension. Differential diagnosis includes chronic hypertension, preeclampsia, and gestational hypertension. The patient and her fetus warrant close monitoring throughout the pregnancy for evidence of the evolution of preeclampsia. Blood pressure should be treated with methyldopa or labetalol if it rises >160/100 mmHg.

Discussion: Elevations in blood pressure before 20 weeks' gestation most commonly are due to chronic hypertension. After 20 weeks' gestation, the differential diagnosis must include **preeclampsia** and gestational hypertension. Because most of the morbidity associated with hypertension in pregnancy is due to preeclampsia, a high index of suspicion needs to be maintained for this diagnosis. Symptoms of preeclampsia include headache, visual scintillations and scotomas, and epigastric pain (see Table). Signs of preeclampsia include epigastric tenderness (owing to hepatic congestion) and clonus. Edema is seen commonly in preeclampsia but lacks specificity because it is common in normal pregnancies as well. Laboratory manifestations of preeclampsia include an elevated creatinine, thrombocytopenia, elevated AST, elevated uric acid, and proteinuria. Whenever blood pressure rises after 20 weeks' gestation, the clinician should review the patient carefully for evidence of any of these features. If any evidence of preeclampsia is found, prompt involvement of an obstetrician is essential. Fetal monitoring needs to be instituted, and decisions regarding outpatient versus inpatient management need to be made. If there is no evidence of preeclampsia at that time, continued vigilance for its subsequent evolution remains essential.

In general, mild-to-moderate hypertension in the absence of preeclampsia represents only a slight increase in risk to mother and fetus, and treatment of blood pressures <160/100 mmHg are not known to confer any advantage to the fetus or mother in the context of pregnancy. If blood pressure rises >160/100 mmHg, the preferred antihypertensives in pregnancy generally are methyldopa and the β-blockers pindolol and labetalol (see Table next page). Angiotensin-converting enzyme (ACE) inhibitors and angiotensin II receptor antagonists should not be used in pregnancy because both types of agents can precipitate renal failure and its complications in the fetus. Use of ACE inhibitors in the early first trimester is not known to have any ill effects, however.

The present patient was admitted to the hospital for observation, fetal evaluation, and a 24-hour urine for protein. All findings were normal, and her blood pressure remained elevated but stayed <160/100 mmHg, so no medication was initiated. She was discharged to close follow-up with regular fetal monitoring. Three weeks later, the patient developed a severe headache with visual scintillations and was admitted to the hospital with a blood pressure of 165/100. Her preeclampsia laboratory tests revealed a uric acid of 6.2 mg/dL, 3+ proteinuria, and a slightly elevated AST. Labor was induced for preeclampsia, and she delivered a vigorous 36-week infant within 12 hours of admission. By 6 weeks postpartum, her blood pressure was consistently <140/85 mmHg without any treatment.

Manifestations of Preeclampsia

Symptoms
  Headache
  Visual scintillations and scotoma
  Epigastric pain
Signs
  Retinal arteriolar vasospasm
  Epigastric tenderness
  Edema (common also in normal pregnancies)
  Clonus
  Less commonly, seizure and pulmonary edema
Common laboratory manifestations
  Proteinuria >300 mg/24 h
  ↑ Creatinine
  ↑ Uric acid
  ↑ Aspartate aminotransferase
  ↓ Platelets

Agent	Dosage	Benefits	Side Effects
Methyldopa	250–500 mg bid–qid (maximum 3000 mg/d)	FDA pregnancy classification B Agent most extensively studied for use in pregnancy	Commonly: maternal somnolence, dry mouth Rarely: hemolytic anemia, hepatitis, depression 15% of women do not tolerate the doses of this medication necessary to control blood pressure
Labetalol	100–600 mg bid-tid (maximum 2400 mg/d)	FDA pregnancy classification B Seems to be less risk of fetal growth restriction than may occur with pure β-blockers	Scalp tingling, tremulousness, headache, hepatotoxicity, possibly small-for-gestation-age infants TID dosing may be necessary due to altered pharmokinetics of this agent in pregnancy.
Pindolol	5–15 mg BID (maximum 60 mg/day)	FDA pregnancy classification B Probably preferred agent among β-blockers because of intrinsic sympathomimetic activity.	Small-for-gestational-age infants (especially if used throughout gestation), neonatal bradycardia, and hypoglycemia all have been reported with other β-blockers and may occur with pindolol

FDA, Food and Drug Administration; bid, twice a day; qid, four times a day; tid, three times a day.

Clinical Pearls

1. Hypertension presenting in pregnancy before 20 weeks' gestation almost always is due to chronic hypertension. After 20 weeks, careful, regular consideration of the possible diagnosis of preeclampsia must occur.

2. Treatment of blood pressures <160/100 mmHg in pregnancy is not necessary. If treatment is deemed appropriate, methyldopa, pindolol, or labetalol can be used. Use of ACE inhibitors or angiotensin II receptor blockers should be avoided in pregnancy.

3. Severe hypertension (>180/105 to 180/110 or any elevation of blood pressure with evidence of acute target organ damage) in pregnancy can be managed acutely with intravenous labetalol or hydralazine.

REFERENCES

1. ACOG technical bulletin: Hypertension in pregnancy. No. 219, January 1996 (replaces no. 91, February 1986). Int J Gynaecol Obstet 53:175–183, 1996.
2. Sibai BM: Drug therapy: Treatment of hypertension in pregnant women. N Engl J Med 335:257–265, 1996.
3. Rey E, LeLorier J, Burgess E, et al: Report of the Canadian Hypertension Society Consensus Conference: Pharmacologic management of hypertensive disorders in pregnancy. Can Med Assoc J 157:907–919, 1997.
4. Ferrer RL, Chiquette E, Stevens KR, et al: Evidence Report on Management of Chronic Hypertension During Pregnancy. Agency for Health Care Policy and Research, 1999.
5. Magee LA, Ornstein MP, von Dadelszen P: Fortnightly review: Management of hypertension in pregnancy. BMJ 318:1332–1336, 1999.

PATIENT 43

A 20-year-old pregnant woman with epigastric
pain and elevated hepatic transaminases

A 20-year-old gravida 1, para 0 pregnant woman at 37 weeks' gestation who has had no previous significant medical history presents with a 24-hour history of epigastric pain and a mild throbbing bitemporal headache. She denies nausea, vomiting, change in bowel movements, fever and chills, or visual changes.

Physical Examination: Temperature 98.7°F, pulse 94, respirations 14, blood pressure 145/90. Patient appears to be in no distress. Skin: no jaundice. HEENT: normal funduscopic examination, no sinus tenderness, no neck stiffness. Chest: normal. Cardiac: normal heart sounds, but a nonradiating grade III/VI ejection systolic murmur is heard at the left upper sternal border. Abdomen: moderate epigastric tenderness but negative Murphy's sign. Extremities: mild bilateral peripheral lower limb edema. Neuromuscular: brisk reflexes but no clonus.

Laboratory Findings: CBC: WBC 7600/μL with a normal differential, hemoglobin 14 g/dL, platelets 92,000/μL. Creatinine 1.1 mg/dL (normal in pregnancy is <0.8 mg/dL) Uric acid 5.6 mg/dL (normal in pregnancy is <5.0 mg/dL). Aspartate aminotransferase 130 U/L. Urinalysis: 3+ proteinuria. ECG: normal.

Questions: What are the possible explanations for this patient's constellation of findings? How would you manage her at this time?

Diagnosis and Treatment: Probable HELLP (*h*emolysis, *e*levated *l*iver enzymes, *l*ow *p*latelets) syndrome with differential diagnosis including gallbladder disease, infectious hepatitis, and acute fatty liver of pregnancy. In this case, the elevated blood pressure and proteinuria suggest preeclampsia, and because the patient is at 37 weeks' gestation, she should be delivered.

Discussion: The most important causes of pregnancy-related hepatic disease in the third trimester are preeclampsia and HELLP syndrome, acute fatty liver of pregnancy, and cholestasis of pregnancy (see Table). Other causes of liver disease commonly occurring in pregnancy are acute viral hepatitis, biliary disease, drug-induced hepatitis, and alcohol effects. Acute viral hepatitis usually is associated with fever and an exposure history, and the alanine aminotransferase value is usually in the thousands. Biliary disease is relatively common in pregnancy and usually presents with colicky right upper quadrant pain in association with an elevated alkaline phosphatase, γ-glutamyltransferase, and bilirubin and biliary stones on ultrasound. The alkaline phosphatase level is increased twofold in the normal pregnancy as a result of placental production of this enzyme. It is always worth considering medication as a possible cause of elevated liver enzymes during pregnancy; in particular, nitrofurantoin, methyldopa, and labetalol (all of which commonly are prescribed by obstetricians) can cause significant hepatic necrosis. Alcoholic hepatitis is another important and common cause to be considered. Finally, because many women enter the health care system for the first time when they are pregnant, the clinician should consider the possibility that a liver enzyme abnormality identified during pregnancy may not be a new problem but rather can represent a previously undiagnosed chronic problem, such as chronic hepatitis B or C or autoimmune hepatitis.

In the present patient, the presence of proteinuria and hypertension makes preeclampsia the most likely diagnosis. A peripheral smear confirmed the presence of fragmented RBCs, and lactate dehydrogenase was found to be

Important Pregnancy-Related Causes of Hepatic Disease Presenting in the Third Trimester

Diagnosis	Features	Treatment
Preeclampsia/ HELLP syndrome	A complication of severe preeclampsia, so hypertension or proteinuria or both are usually present Occurs in 0.1% of pregnancies but in 4% to 12% of cases of severe preeclampsia ALT usually <500 U/L Platelets <100,000/µL Fragmented RBCs on smear and elevated lactate dehydrogenase	Delivery with close monitoring
Acute fatty liver of pregnancy	Occurs in 0.008% of pregnancies Viral-like malaise, nausea and vomiting, and epigastric or right upper quadrant tenderness are typical presenting features ALT 100–500 U/L Hypoglycemia may occur Significant risk of maternal mortality	Delivery with close monitoring Screen newborn for LCHAD deficiency because acute fatty liver of pregnancy is associated with the presence of this inborn error of metabolism in the newborn
Cholestasis of pregnancy	Occurs in 0.1% to 0.2% of pregnancies in the United States but is much more common in Chile and Scandinavian countries Presents as severe, generalized pruritus Serum bile acids markedly elevated, but bilirubin, ALT, and alkaline phosphatase are usually normal or only mildly increased	Increased monitoring of fetus and consideration of delivery with lung maturation around 34 weeks because some evidence exists that the fetus is at increased risk of sudden unexplained death Symptomatic relief may be obtained with cholestyramine or ursodeoxycholic acid.

ALT, alanine aminotransferase; LCHAD, long-chain 3-hydroxyacyl coenzyme A dehydrogenase.

markedly elevated, confirming the diagnosis of HELLP syndrome. Labor was induced with cervical dinoprostone (Prostin) and intravenous oxytocin (Pitocin), and CBC, liver enzymes, and creatinine were followed every 6 hours. The patient was placed on magnesium to prevent eclamptic seizures. She delivered a healthy 2.5-kg boy within 24 hours. Postpartum, her laboratory values normalized over the following 72 hours.

Clinical Pearls

1. After 20 weeks' gestation, preeclampsia always should be considered in the differential diagnosis of elevated liver enzymes in pregnancy. Accompanying findings of new-onset hypertension and proteinuria make this diagnosis likely. If there is associated thrombocytopenia and evidence of hemolysis, the diagnosis of HELLP syndrome can be made.

2. Progressive elevation in liver enzymes toward term, in association with jaundice, fever, and hypoglycemia, makes the diagnosis of acute fatty liver of pregnancy likely. This diagnosis is life-threatening and requires delivery as soon as possible. Screening the newborn for errors in fatty acid oxidation (specifically LCHAD deficiency) is essential.

3. Cholestasis of pregnancy presents as severe pruritus and can cause mild elevations in liver enzymes. Because of an association between this entity and sudden fetal death, many experts advocate for early delivery of women with this condition.

REFERENCES

1. Reyes H: The spectrum of liver and gastrointestinal disease seen in cholestasis of pregnancy. Gastroenterol Clin North Am 21:905–921, 1992.
2. Bacq Y, Riely CA: Acute fatty liver of pregnancy: The hepatologist's view. Gastroenterologist 1:257–264, 1993.
3. Knox TA, Olans LB: Liver disease in pregnancy. N Engl J Med 335:569–576, 1996.
4. Ibdah JA, Bennett MJ, Rinaldo P, et al: A fetal fatty-acid oxidation disorder as a cause of liver disease in pregnant women. N Engl J Med 340:1723–1731, 1999.

PATIENT 44

A 35-year-old man with postoperative excessive urine output

A 35-year-old man with Cushing's disease undergoes transsphenoidal surgery for resection of a pituitary adenoma. One day after surgery, he experiences an abrupt increase in urine output (range, 280–300 mL/h).

Physical Examination: Temperature 98.6°F, pulse 110, respirations 16, blood pressure 96/52. HEENT: cushingoid facial appearance. Chest: clear. Cardiac: normal S_1 and S_2 with no murmurs or gallops. Back: *buffalo hump* present. Abdomen: obese, soft, nontender, no masses. Striae present in the lower quadrants.

Laboratory Findings: Serum sodium 160 mEq/L, serum osmolality 330 mOsm/kg. Urine specific gravity 1.004, urine osmolality 52 mOsm/kg.

Question: What is the diagnosis?

Diagnosis: Postoperative diabetes insipidus (DI).

Discussion: DI is defined as polyuria of 2–10 L/day with dilute urine (specific gravity 1.000–1.005) in conjunction with high serum osmolality (>295 mOsm/kg) and high serum sodium (>145 mEq/L). Patients who are awake also complain of thirst and polydipsia. In the perioperative patient, DI occurs with head trauma or neurosurgery, especially surgery involving the pituitary or hypothalamus. Other causes are listed in the Table below. The condition is generally temporary as long as the hypothalamic-hypophyseal tract has remained intact. Permanent DI can result, however, if >85% of neurons in the supraoptic and paraventricular nuclei are destroyed. DI is common in patients who have undergone transsphenoidal surgery (occurring in approximately 30% of patients) and is believed to be due to neuronal shock. It generally occurs abruptly during the first postoperative day and resolves within 2 to 5 days.

Causes of Central Diabetes Insipidus

Neurosurgery (especially pituitary or
   hypothalamic)
Brain tumor
Head trauma
Generalized trauma
Central nervous system infection
Cerebral edema
Medications (morphine, reserpine, phenytoin,
   chlorpromazine)
Idiopathic

In many cases, postoperative DI can be managed with increased intravenous and oral fluids without the addition of vasopressin. Daily fluid replacement must take into account insensible losses in addition to the large urine output. The hourly intravenous rate should include the hourly fluid needs for the clinical situation (i.e., the patient's metabolic needs and insensible losses) and the amount of urine output produced in the previous hour. When medication is necessary, aqueous vasopressin has a short duration of action and so can be used in the acute setting, such as trauma or neurosurgery, when function is expected to return within a few days. It is thus easier to watch for the return of neurohypophyseal function and prevent water intoxication in patients who are receiving large amounts of intravenous fluids. Aqueous vasopressin can have pressor effects; when this is undesirable, desmopressin acetate (DDAVP), a synthetic vasopressin, should be used instead (because it has no pressor effects). DDAVP can be given intravenously twice a day in the immediate postoperative period or in patients who are not conscious, then changed to the intranasal form when patients are alert and awake.

For patients with residual DI manifested by mild polyuria, oral medications that stimulate antidiuretic hormone release are available (Table below). During the acute phase or for patients with permanent damage, vasopressin or desmopressin should be used.

It is rare for nephrogenic DI to occur *de novo* postoperatively; it generally is seen in patients who already have DI preoperatively. For intraoperative management of patients with preexisting nephrogenic DI, the anesthesiologist should consider central venous pressure monitoring to guide fluid management because the urine output remains elevated even with volume depletion, and serum sodium and serum osmolality should be checked frequently.

The present patient received vigorous fluid repletion with normal saline initially because tachycardia and hypotension reflected intravascular fluid depletion. When his hemodynamics were stable, he received a 5% dextrose solution at an hourly rate that replaced insensible losses and the

Pharmacologic Agents for Treating
Diabetes Insipidus

Agent	Dosing
Mild polyuria	
Carbamazepine	200 mg 2–3 times/d
Chlorpropamide	200–500 mg/d
Clofibrate	500 mg 4 times/d
Moderate-to-severe polyuria	
Aqueous vasopression (Pitressin)	5–10 U subcutaneously every 3–8 h
Desmopression (DDAVP)	5–10 μg every 12–24 h intravenously
Lypressin (Diapid)	2–4 U every 4–6 h intravenously
Vasopressin tannate in oil (Pitressin)	5 U intramuscularly every 24–72 h

previous hour's urinary losses. Aqueous vaso-pressin was started, with rapid results. Urine output decreased to 150 mL/h in the first hour after receiving 5 U of vasopressin subcutaneously. The dosing interval was titrated to the patient's response (5 U every 5–6 hours). On the fourth postoperative day, because his hypothalamic hypophyseal functioning was expected to improve soon, the vasopressin was given only when urine output started to increase. The vasopressin requirement dropped dramatically by the fifth postoperative day, and the patient was able to maintain appropriate water balance. The rest of his recovery was uneventful.

Clinical Pearls

1. The operative mortality for transsphenoidal surgery is low (approximately 1%), and major morbidity occurs at a rate of 3.4%.

2. The types of major morbidity that occur include hemorrhagic and thrombotic stroke, visual loss, cerebrospinal fluid rhinorrhea, third nerve palsies and sixth nerve palsies, meningitis, and sellar abscess.

3. The initial postoperative remission rate for pituitary adrenocorticotropic hormone adenomas is 91% for microadenomas and 56% for macroadenomas.

REFERENCES

1. Germon K: Fluid and electrolyte problems associated with diabetes insipidus and syndrome of inappropriate antidiuretic hormone. Nursing Clin North Am 22:785–796, 1987.
2. Mathes DD: Management of common endocrine disorders. In Stone DJ, Bogdonoff DL, Leisure GS, et al (eds): Perioperative Care. St Louis, Mosby, 1998, pp 248–250.
3. Laws ER, Thapar K: Pituitary surgery. Endocrinol Metab Clin North Am 28:119–132, 1999.
4. Shaw RJ: Aquaporins and the surgeon: Cautionary tales. J R Coll Surg Edin 46:237–239, 2001.

PATIENT 45

A 78-year-old man with a history of deep venous thrombosis awaiting total knee replacement

A 78-year-old man with severe degenerative joint disease is awaiting left total knee replacement. Six months previously, he underwent right total knee replacement. He tolerated the procedure well but developed a deep venous thrombosis (DVT) of the right popliteal vein postoperatively despite use of warfarin (Coumadin) and pneumatic compression sleeves. His international normalized ratio (INR) was not therapeutic until the fourth postoperative day, however. He has no history of DVTs earlier in his life and has no family history of DVT.

Physical Examination: Pulse 74, blood pressure 144/86. General appearance: Elderly man in distress when walking secondary to knee pain. Chest: clear. Heart: regular rate and rhythm. No murmur, rub, or gallop. Abdomen: benign. Neurologic: benign. Extremities: trace pretibial edema.

Laboratory Findings: Electrolytes, chemistries, and CBC all within normal limits.

Question: What clinical factors constitute high risk for postoperative DVT?

Answer: Total joint replacement of the hip and knee and other orthopedic surgeries place patients at the highest risk for postoperative DVT. Some other clinical factors placing patients at high risk are gynecologic surgery for malignancy, prior DVT, hypercoagulable states, and spinal cord injury.

Discussion: Current accepted therapies for DVT prophylaxis for orthopedic procedures include low-molecular-weight heparin, adjusted-dose unfractionated heparin, warfarin, and pneumatic compression devices. Pneumatic compression devices are believed to be inferior to the other listed methods, and although they can be used alone, it is recommended that another modality, such as low-molecular-weight heparin, be added after 48 hours postoperatively. Adjusted-dose unfractionated heparin is an acceptable method of prophylaxis but requires multiple laboratory evaluations for titration of the activated partial thromboplastin time and is inconvenient to the patient and the physician.

Low-molecular-weight heparin and adjusted-dose warfarin currently are the most commonly used modalities for postoperative venous thromboembolism prophylaxis; there are pros and cons to the use of each. The low-molecular-weight heparins have the convenience of no requirement for associated laboratory monitoring, but they are expensive and not covered by all types of insurance. The low-molecular-weight heparins also have the benefit of providing anticoagulation starting a few hours after the first dose, which warfarin does not. If there is postoperative bleeding, however, it is more difficult to reverse: Although vitamin K and fresh frozen plasma can counteract warfarin, protamine must be used for low-molecular-weight heparin, and it works incompletely. (It neutralizes all of the anti–factor IIa activity of low-molecular-weight heparin but only about 60% of the anti–factor Xa activity). Warfarin is inexpensive and reversed fairly readily, but it often does not reach therapeutic effect postoperatively for a few days. Warfarin and the low-molecular-weight heparins have been shown to reduce the overall risk of venous thrombotic events significantly in lower extremity total joint replacement.

The rate of DVT and pulmonary embolism for patients undergoing hip and knee replacement and repair of hip fracture without prophylaxis are shown in the Table at top right. The reduction in DVT afforded by warfarin and enoxaparin for total knee replacement and the associated rates of major bleeding caused by those therapies are shown in the Table at right. It has been made a priority to improve these statistics further by exploring new clinical alternatives.

Rates of Deep Venous Thrombosis
Without Prophylaxis

Hip fracture	36–60%
Total hip replacement	45–57%
Total knee replacement	40–84%

A new pentasaccharide compound, fondaparinux sodium, has finished phase III clinical trials for the prevention of DVT after orthopedic surgery and is newly available for clinical use. This medication is a synthetic indirect factor Xa inhibitor that structurally resembles the antithrombin binding site of heparin. It does not prolong the activated partial thromboplastin time or the activated coagulation time. Clinically important bleeding occurred at a frequency similar to low-molecular-weight heparin in clinical trials. Four large randomized, double-blind studies showed greater efficacy than low-molecular-weight heparin when used after hip and knee replacement surgery.

Another new compound, ximelagatran, is a direct thrombin inhibitor currently undergoing phase III clinical trials for the prevention of DVT in postoperative orthopedic patients. ximelagatran is an oral prodrug that is metabolized to the active metabolite melagatran. A study showed that the rates of postoperative DVT and pulmonary embolism in the Ximelagatran patient group did not differ significantly from the enoxaparin group, and there was no major bleeding in the ximelagatran group.

The present patient was thought to be at high risk for postoperative DVT because of a history of prior postoperative DVT and the nature of this surgery. The fact that the patient did not have a therapeutic INR until postoperative day 4 with his prior surgery was thought to play a role in the occurrence of the

Rates of Deep Venous Thrombosis in Total
Knee Replacement With Warfarin and
Enoxaparin

	Warfarin	Enoxaparin
Distal DVT	59%	38%
Proximal DVT	13%	3%
Major bleeding	2%	5%

DVT, deep venous thrombosis.

DVT. For his upcoming surgery, it was decided to place him on postoperative low-molecular-weight heparin, which begins to act 4 to 5 hours after the first dose. If the patient truly had been an **anticoagulation failure** (development of a DVT despite full anticoagulation postoperatively), he would have needed to be evaluated for an inferior vena caval filter. On availability of newer agents, the patient may be an excellent candidate for a pentasaccharide compound or a direct thrombin inhibitor.

Clinical Pearls

1. One physiologic reason that hip surgery creates such a high risk for DVT is that the femoral vein is compressed intraoperatively because of the surgical technique.

2. Pentasaccharides will likely be acceptable therapy for patients with heparin-induced thrombocytopenia and may be appropriate for routine postoperative DVT prophylaxis.

3. A recent study showed the rate of DVT after major knee surgery to be 12.5% with fondaparinux (a pentasaccharide) and 27.8% with enoxaparin.

REFERENCES

1. Spiro TE, Johnson GJ, Christie MJ, for the Enoxaparin Clinical Trial Group: Efficacy and safety of enoxaparin to prevent deep venous thrombosis after hip replacement surgery. Ann Intern Med 121:81–89, 1994.
2. Leclerc JR, Geerts WH, Desjardins L, et al: Prevention of venous thromboembolism (VTE) after knee arthroplasty: A randomized double-blind trial comparing enoxaparin with warfarin sodium. Ann Intern Med 124:619–626, 1996.
3. Heiut JA, Colwell CW, Francis CW, et al: Comparison of the oral direct thrombin inhibitor Ximelagatran with enoxaparin as prophylaxis against venous thromboembolism after total hip replacement. Arch Intern Med 161:2215–2221, 2001.
4. Hirsh J: New anticoagulants. Am Heart J 142 (pt 2):S3–S8, 2001.
5. Bauer KA, Eriksson BI, Lassen MR, et al: Fondaparinux compared with enoxaparin for the prevention of venous thromboembolism after elective major knee surgery. N Engl J Med 345:1305–1310, 2001.
6. Turpie AG, Gallus AS, Hoek JA: A synthetic pentasaccharide for the prevention of deep vein thrombosis after total hip replacement. N Engl J Med 344:619–625, 2001.
7. Rai R, Sprengler A, Elrod KC, Young WB: Perspectives on factor Xa inhibition. Curr Med Chem 8:101–119, 2001.

PATIENT 46

A 77-year-old man with postoperative confusion and agitation

A 77-year-old man underwent repair of a large ventral hernia. His past medical history is notable for mild memory impairment, hypertension, mild chronic obstructive pulmonary disease, and gastroesophageal reflux. On awakening from surgery, the patient is noted to be somnolent and confused to time and place. After awakening further, he remains confused and becomes agitated. He pulls out his intravenous line and his Foley catheter and thinks he was in prison, despite frequent redirecting. He receives 2 mg of haloperidol intramuscularly, which makes him somnolent but does not reduce his confusion. He remains agitated and confused when not on haloperidol. He requires 2 to 3 mg of morphine sulfate intravenously every 6 hours for pain control. In addition to the haloperidol and morphine, his medications include an oral inhalation aerosol (Combivent), metoclopramide, verapamil, and omeprazole.

Physical Examination: Temperature 99.9°F, pulse 100, respirations 16, blood pressure 158/96. General appearance: agitated and oriented to person only, requiring wrist restraints. Oxygen saturation 93% on 2 L of oxygen. Chest: decreased breath sounds throughout, with prolonged expiratory phase but no wheezes or rales. Heart: normal S_1 and S_2. Regular rhythm. No murmur. Abdomen: soft, no masses, hypoactive bowel sounds. Surgical wound intact and dry. Tender at surgical site only.

Laboratory Findings: WBC 10,200/μL, hematocrit 25.2%, platelets 210,000/μL. Sodium 135 mEq/dL, potassium 3.9 mEq/dL, bicarbonate 26 mEq/dL, BUN 19 mg/dL, creatinine 1.3 mg/dL, calcium 9.2 mg/dL, phosphate 3.0 mg/dL, magnesium 1.9 mg/dL. ABG: pH 7.38, PCO_2 43 mmHg, PO_2 75 mmHg. Chest radiograph: depressed diaphragms, hyperinflated lungs consistent with chronic obstructive pulmonary disease. No infiltrates. ECG: sinus rhythm with no ischemic changes.

Question: What is the cause of the patient's postoperative delirium?

Diagnosis: Multifactorial postoperative delirium in a geriatric patient.

Discussion: Delirium is defined as a fluctuation level of consciousness associated with confusion and inattention. **Postoperative delirium** refers to the presence of delirium within 30 days after surgery. The possible causes of delirium are many (Table below). Multiple studies have been performed in the perioperative setting to evaluate which factors predispose patients to postoperative delirium. The main factors that have been identified include use of five or more drugs postoperatively, use of preoperative anticholinergics, preexisting dementia, severe medical illness, and advanced age.

Causes of Postoperative Delirium

Cardiac
   Postoperative myocardial infarction
   Decreases in perfusion owing to congestive
      heart failure, dysrhythmias
Pulmonary
   Hypoxia
   Pneumonia
   Pulmonary embolism
   Fat emboli syndrome
Metabolic
   Hyponatremia/hypernatremia
   Acid-base disturbances
   Hepatic encephalopathy
   Wernicke's encephalopathy
Endocrine
   Hypoglycemia/hyperglycemia
   Hypothyroidism/hyperthyroidism
Neurologic
   Cerebrovascular accident
   Underlying dementia
   Postoperative seizure
   Subarachnoid hemorrhage
Medications
   Anesthetic agents
   Narcotics
   Anticholinergic agents
   Steroids
   Sedatives
   NSAIDs
   Anticonvulsants
   Anti-Parkinson agents
   Lithium
   Cimetidine
   Atropine
   Clonidine
   Antipsychotics
   Digitalis

NSAIDs, nonsteroidal anti-inflammatory drugs.

Marcantonio et al developed a "clinical prediction rule" for predicting postoperative delirium. They found seven preoperative clinical characteristics to be independent correlates of postoperative delirium: age ≥70 years; self-reported alcohol abuse; poor cognitive status; poor functional status; markedly abnormal preoperative serum sodium, potassium, or glucose level; noncardiac thoracic surgery; and aortic aneurysm surgery. Each clinical characteristic present in a given patient earned 1 point except aortic aneurysm surgery, which earned 2 points. Patients with 0 points had a 2% risk of delirium, patients with 1 to 2 points had an 11% risk of delirium, and patients with ≥3 points had a 50% risk of delirium.

This scale is useful in evaluating the preoperative factors that may leave a patient vulnerable to developing postoperative delirium, but it does not take into account possible intraoperative factors that can cause delirium. The study also found that patients who developed delirium had higher rates of major complications, longer lengths of stay, and a higher risk of discharge to either rehabilitative or long-term care facilities.

A subsequent study by Marcantonio et al looked at intraoperative factors associated with postoperative delirium. They found that delirium was related to greater intraoperative blood loss, more postoperative blood transfusions, and a postoperative hematocrit of <30%. The method of anesthesia and intraoperative hemodynamic complications were not found to be associated factors, although other studies have found that perioperative hypotension does correlate with postoperative delirium.

Certain types of surgery have been associated with delirium. Cardiac surgery can cause cerebral ischemia through hypoperfusion and microemboli. Hip fracture repair has a reported prevalence of delirium of 9.5% to 19%. Important causes have been found to be advanced age, preexisting dementia, environmental settings, infection, fluid and electrolyte abnormalities, and perioperative medications. Cataract surgery also is associated with delirium because of visual loss and the use of ophthalmologic medications with anticholinergic properties.

In identifying delirium, physicians can use a modified mini-mental status examination (Table, next page) in addition to observation of level of consciousness. When identified, the underlying cause must be sought and corrected. Postoperative delirium often has multiple causes. The patient should undergo a physical examination; an ECG and cardiac enzymes should be considered to rule out a silent postoperative myocardial infarction.

Bedside Tests of Mental Status	
Test	Function
Name, month, year	Orientation
Spell "world" backwards	Attention
Current events	General knowledge
Recall 3 objects at 5 minutes	Short-term memory
Comparing common objects	Abstract reasoning
Subtract serial 7s	Calculation

Basic laboratory tests, such as electrolytes, divalents, and a CBC, should be ordered. The medication regimen should be evaluated and simplified as much as possible. Other tests may be ordered according to the clinical situation. Diagnoses such as **ICU psychosis** and **sundowning** should be used only when all clinical entities have been ruled out.

Neuroleptic medications, such as haloperidol and risperidone, are used most commonly for psychotic symptoms and agitation. Risperidone has a better side-effect profile than haloperidol, but it cannot be given intramuscularly or intravenously (haloperidol can). For faster onset of action, haloperidol should be used. Olanzapine has the lowest occurrence of extrapyramidal side effects and can also be used, especially for patients with Parkinson's disease. Although benzodiazepines are useful to help decrease agitation and reduce the extrapyramidal side effects of the antipsychotics, they can be oversedating, especially in the elderly, and can cause respiratory depression and hypotension. For elderly patients who require treatment for agitation who cannot use antipsychotics at all, small scheduled doses of trazodone, starting at 12.5 mg every 8 to 12 hours, can be tried.

The present patient was believed to have multifactorial postoperative delirium. His age was >70 years, he lost a significant amount of blood, and he had a postoperative hematocrit of 25%. In addition, he required morphine for pain control and was receiving metoclopramide, an anticholinergic, for gastroesophageal reflux disease symptoms and postoperative nausea. His postoperative ECG revealed 1-mm ST depression in leads V5 and V6, and troponin was 5.8, indicating a silent postoperative non–Q wave myocardial infarction. The metoclopramide was stopped, the pain medication was minimized, he received 2 U of packed red blood cells, and he received medication for his postoperative myocardial infarction (aspirin, atenolol, and nitropaste). The patient was reoriented frequently and received 1.0 mg of risperidone twice a day. His delirium improved over the following 3 days, although he still was having some episodes of mild confusion in the evenings, and he required transfer to a long-term care facility.

Clinical Pearls

1. It is important to differentiate delirium from dementia, although demented patients also are at risk for developing postoperative delirium.

2. Some hip fracture patients develop delirium preoperatively, likely because of the combination of trauma, pain, and abrupt transfer to the hospital. The reason for their fall should be sought to rule out new underlying medical illness.

3. Trials are under way to evaluate if donepezil (Aricept) can decrease postoperative confusion.

REFERENCES
1. Marcantonio ER, Goldman L, Magione CM, et al: A clinical prediction rule for delirium after elective non cardiac surgery. JAMA 271:134–139, 1994.
2. Dyer CB, Ashton CM, Teasdale TA: Postoperative delirium. Arch Intern Med 155:461–465, 1995.
3. Marcantonio ER, Goldman L, Orav EJ, et al: The association of intraoperative factors with the development of postoperative delirium. Am J Med 105:380–384, 1998.
4. Edlund A, Lundstrom M, Brannstrom B, et al: Delirium before and after operation for femoral neck fracture. J Am Geriatr Soc 49:1335–1340, 2001.
5. Winawer N: Postoperative delirium. Med Clin North Am 85:1229–1239, 2001.

PATIENT 47

A 27-year-old pregnant patient with fever, nausea, and abdominal pain

A 27-year-old pregnant patient at 25 weeks' gestation presents with a 1-day history of fever, nausea, vomiting, and worsening right lower quadrant pain.

Physical Examination: Temperature 101.7°F, pulse 102, respirations 20, blood pressure 106/68. HEENT: normal. Chest: clear. Heart: regular rate and rhythm. Grade II/VI systolic flow murmur in the left upper sternal border without radiation. Abdomen: gravid fundus at 2 cm above the umbilicus. Hypoactive bowel sounds. Tenderness of the right lower quadrant without rebound. Extremities: trace pretibial edema.

Laboratory Findings: WBC 15,600/μL, bands 13%, polymorphonuclear neutrophils 80%, lymphocytes 7%, hematocrit 32.2%, platelets 213,000 μL. Electrolytes: normal. Aspartate transaminase 51 mg/dL, alanine transaminase 45 mg/dL, total bilirubin 0.9 mg/dL, alkaline phosphatase 402 mg/dL.

Questions: What is the most likely diagnosis? What are the problems associated with surgery during pregnancy?

Diagnosis: Appendicitis in a pregnant patient.

Discussion: Acute appendicitis is the most common indication for surgery in pregnancy. It occurs most commonly in the second trimester, with an incidence of approximately 30% in the first trimester, 45% in the second trimester, and 25% in the third trimester. Making the diagnosis during pregnancy may be clouded by the fact that some signs and symptoms of normal pregnancy also are symptoms of appendicitis, such as nausea, vomiting, leukocytosis, and anorexia. Delay in diagnosis and treatment can result in an increase in maternal and fetal morbidity and mortality.

Diagnosis can be difficult, although there have been reports that helical CT is safe and effective. Since 1932, the prevailing thought regarding appendicitis in pregnancy has been that the change in position of the appendix would cause a change in the location of pain toward the right upper quadrant as pregnancy progresses. In 1932, Baer et al conducted barium studies on 78 pregnant women that showed the enlarging uterus pushes the appendix upward. A more recent review of 67 cases of appendicitis revealed, however, that the most common presenting symptom regardless of gestational age was pain the right *lower* quadrant, not the right upper quadrant. Pain in the right upper quadrant was seen occasionally, as was pain in the left lower quadrant, midabdomen, epigastrium, or a combination of these.

Regarding **surgical approach,** laparoscopic surgery now is being performed successfully during pregnancy for a variety of intra-abdominal conditions, including appendicitis. Currently the most commonly performed laparoscopic surgery in pregnancy is cholecystectomy. Although laparoscopic surgery offers the advantages of less postoperative pain, less postoperative ileus, and shorter length of hospital stay, there are several disadvantages in pregnant patients: The pneumoperitoneum induced by carbon dioxide (CO_2) insufflation further limits diaphragmatic expansion, which already has been affected by the gravid uterus. CO_2 insufflation is associated with an increased peak airway pressure, a further decrease in functional reserve capacity, increased ventilation-perfusion mismatching, and increased alveolar-arterial oxygen gradient. CO_2 insufflation also causes CO_2 absorption across the peritoneum and into the maternal circulation. Elimination of CO_2 depends on an increase in minute ventilation, but mechanical hyperventilation can decrease utero-placental perfusion. Postoperatively the smaller incisions have resulted, however, in less splinting; a decreased degree of postoperative reflex inhibition of diaphragmatic function; and better functional residual capacity, forced expiratory volume in 1 second, forced vital capacity, PO_2, and PCO_2 measurements compared with conventional laparotomy patients.

Although there have been fetal deaths associated with laparoscopic surgery, several small studies have shown comparable outcomes between laparoscopy and laparotomy groups. A new type of laparoscopic surgery uses mechanical lifting of the abdominal wall instead of CO_2 insufflation. This gasless approach may cause fewer hemodynamic changes.

The physiologic changes induced by pregnancy have a significant impact on management of surgery and anesthesia. Anesthetic and surgical treatments must take into account the mother and the fetus. Starting at about 18 to 22 weeks, women in the supine position can experience aortocaval compression from the enlarging uterus. Lateral positioning is important. Also, pregnancy causes a decrease in anesthetic requirements. The patient may be more sensitive to axonal block by local anesthetic, and during general anesthesia, the minimal alveolar concentration decreases. Pregnant patients are at a greater risk for aspiration because of decreased gastroesophageal sphincter tone. Several pulmonary changes in pregnancy affect intraoperative management. Because the residual volume and functional residual capacity decrease and because minute ventilation and oxygen consumption increase, the overall oxygen reserve in pregnant women decreases. Pregnant patients develop hypoxia and hypercapnia more quickly with hypoventilation or apnea.

A central issue in caring for pregnant patients is the maintenance of placental blood flow. In the case of maternal hypotension, initial treatments consist of lateral maternal positioning (to displace the uterus laterally off the aorta and vena cava), fluid boluses, Trendelenburg position, and use of compression stockings. If pressors are necessary, medications such as dopamine, epinephrine, and α-adrenergic agents should not be used because they can decrease uterine blood flow. Ephedrine can be used, as can small doses of phenylephrine. Administration of oxygen to the mother improves fetal oxygenation, but because fetal oxygen tension does not exceed 65 mmHg, fetal hyperoxia is not a risk.

Regarding the safety of the anesthetic agents, some small retrospective studies have shown a possible association of neural tube defects with first-trimester anesthesia. Larger studies have not been able to identify an increase in any type of congenital anomaly but have reported an increase in miscarriage and low-birth-weight infants. These findings were thought to be due to the underlying diseases that necessitated the surgery. Although there are no known specific teratogenic syndromes caused by anesthetics, many practitioners delay surgery to the second trimester when possible. Neuromuscular blocking agents do not cross the placenta to any clinically significant degree.

The present patient underwent a conventional laparotomy for appendicitis. Her intraoperative course was uncomplicated; she later delivered a healthy infant at 39 weeks' gestation. The mild increase in alkaline phosphatase was consistent with increases seen in normal pregnancy because of placental content of alkaline phosphatase.

Clinical Pearls

1. Acute appendicitis in pregnancy occurs at an incidence of <1% of all pregnancies.
2. The fetal mortality rate in uncomplicated appendicitis is <5%, but rises to almost 30% if perforation occurs.
3. Overall, surgery during the first trimester is associated with a miscarriage rate of 12%. Surgery during the third trimester is associated with a 30% rate of premature labor and early delivery. The second trimester is associated with a miscarriage rate approaching 0%, and the rate of premature labor is <10%. In addition, there is no risk of teratogenesis.
4. Fetal and uterine monitoring should be performed intraoperatively whenever possible.

REFERENCES

1. Baer JL, Reis RA, Araens RA: Appendicitis in pregnancy with changes in position and axis of the normal appendix in pregnancy. JAMA 98, 1932.
2. Gianopoulos JG: Establishing the criteria for anesthesia and other precautions for surgery during pregnancy. Surg Clin North Am 75, 1995.
3. Rosen MA: Management of anesthesia for the pregnant surgical patient. Anesthesiology 91:1159–1163, 1999.
4. Curet MJ: Special problems in laparoscopic surgery. Surg Clin North Am 80:1093–1110, 2000.
5. Mourad J, Elliott JP, Erickson L, Lisboa L: Appendicitis in pregnancy: New information that contradicts long-held clinical beliefs. Am J Obstet Gynecol 182:1027–1029, 2000.
6. Shay DC, Bhavani-Shankar K, Datta S: Laparoscopic surgery during pregnancy. Anesth Clin North Am 19:57–67, 2001.

PATIENT 48

A 55-year-old man with postoperative agitation and hypertension

A 55-year-old man presents after a motor vehicle accident for repair of a fractured humerus and fractured tibia. Preoperatively, he denies any medical problems or use of any medications. Intraoperatively, his blood pressure is labile and responds to small doses of labetalol. Postoperatively, he becomes acutely confused, tremulous, tachycardic, and hypertensive.

Physical Examination: Temperature 99.1°F, pulse 122, respirations 20, blood pressure 178/98 mmHg. HEENT: normal. Chest: clear. Heart: normal. Abdomen: soft, nontender, no hepatosplenomegaly, no ascites.

Laboratory Findings: WBC 4,400/μL, hematocrit 34%, platelets 103,000/μL, mean corpuscular volume 106, sodium 133 mEq/dL, chloride 100 mEq/dL, bicarbonate 23 mEq/L, magnesium 1.1 mEq/dL, phosphorus 2.0 mg/dL, international normalized ratio (INR), 1.4.

Question: What is the cause of the patient's confusion?

Diagnosis: Acute alcohol withdrawal.

Discussion: Usually patients who are alcohol abusers do not identify it to their physicians as a problem when they present for medical care. A high index of suspicion should be maintained. Clues to significant use of alcohol include the presence of macrocytosis and elevations in hepatic enzymes γ-glutamyl transpeptidase, aspartate transaminase, and alanine transaminase. Patients also may have significant decreases in magnesium and phosphorus. If they have not been eating, albumin is decreased, as may be calcium and potassium. If there is significant hepatic damage, this causes a decrease in clotting factors with a subsequent abnormal INR; hepatic damage also decreases serum albumin further.

Signs on physical examination often are not evident until significant hepatic cirrhosis is present. (An exception is the patient with alcoholic hepatitis, who will have an enlarged, tender liver.) The liver should be small and nonpalpable, but the spleen may be enlarged. Ascites and peripheral edema may be present. Skin changes consistent with significant cirrhosis include telangiectasias, spider angiomas, palmar erythema, caput medusa, and jaundice. The present patient was a significant alcohol abuser but did not yet have significant cirrhosis and so did not manifest these telltale physical examination changes, with the exception of a few angiomas.

When hospitalized, alcohol abusers are at risk of developing withdrawal symptoms, termed **alcohol withdrawal syndrome**. Alcohol withdrawal can manifest itself only as mild anxiety or psychomotor agitation; the alcohol withdrawal syndrome presents with more significant symptoms and is defined as two or more of the symptoms or signs shown in the Table. In its worst form, patients develop delirium tremens, which even when treated has a mortality of 5%. Alcohol withdrawal signs and symptoms can begin 6 to 8 hours after the last ingestion. The percentage of alcohol abusers who develop the acute withdrawal syndrome varies greatly from study to study. These patients often escape detection until significant symptoms are present; maintaining a high index of suspicion, especially in trauma cases, is a good rule of thumb.

Acute Alcohol Withdrawal Syndrome

Agitation
Anxiety
Autonomic hyperactivity (hypertension, tachycardia, diaphoresis)
Grand mal seizures
Hand tremors
Hallucinations
Insomnia
Nausea, vomiting

Studies have shown that alcohol abusers have a higher degree of postoperative morbidity; in addition to a high risk of alcohol withdrawal syndrome, they have a greater need for repeat surgery; higher rates of infection, bleeding, and cardiac and respiratory complications, and a longer length of stay.

In determining the severity of alcohol withdrawal, a commonly used tool is the Revised Clinical Institute Withdrawal Assessment for Alcohol (CIWA) scale. The CIWA scale measures presence or absence and degree of severity of all the signs and symptoms of alcohol withdrawal: agitation, anxiety, orientation, nausea and vomiting, tremor, diaphoresis, headache, visual disturbance, auditory disturbance, and tactile disturbance. The treatment doses of benzodiazepine and β-blocker or clonidine can be titrated to effect.

Potential medical problems that are manifestations of long-term alcohol abuse should be kept in mind when caring for the alcoholic patient, including chronic hypertension, gastritis, esophagitis, pancreatitis, vitamin deficiencies, malnutrition, poor wound healing, anemia, leukopenia, thrombocytopenia, peripheral neuropathy, Wernicke's encephalopathy, and cerebellar degeneration. Because severe thiamine deficiency can cause Wernicke's encephalopathy, patients should be given thiamine supplementation, especially before receiving a glucose load (e.g., dextrose in intravenous fluids). Thiamine is a cofactor for a transketolase enzyme in carbohydrate metabolism; giving glucose stimulates the reaction and can deplete the body's last stores of thiamine, precipitating acute Wernicke's encephalopathy. The classic signs consist of ataxia, nystagmus, confusion, and ophthalmoplegia, but only a minority of patients manifest all of these signs. Maintaining a high degree of suspicion and routinely giving thiamine supplementation to these patients is important.

The mainstays of treatment for alcohol withdrawal consist of supportive measures such as a calm environment, appropriate electrolyte and nutritional support, and pharmacologic support for the withdrawal symptoms themselves. Benzodiazepines are used to replace alcohol's inhibitory effect on γ-aminobutyric acid receptors in the brain. They also help control the associated autonomic hyperactivity and alcohol withdrawal seizures. Lorazepam and oxazepam are preferred over diazepam because of their shorter half-life. In addition, they are not metabolized by the hepatic cytochrome P-450 pathway and so are less apt to cause delayed elimination in patients with significant hepatic cirrhosis. Studies have shown that dosing benzodiazepines based on symptoms rather than using fixed dosing may result in less sedation and shorter length of stay.

β-Blockers and clonidine (an α-adrenergic blocker) decrease the autonomic hyperactivity seen in alcohol withdrawal. The medications can be titrated as needed to control systemic hypertension, tachycardia, and tremor often seen in alcohol withdrawal. They should not be used without a benzodiazepine, however, because they do not protect against central nervous system signs and symptoms, such as seizures, anxiety, and hallucinations.

Delirium tremens is the most serious form of alcohol withdrawal and generally occurs 2 to 7 days after cessation of alcohol intake. The prevalence is approximately 5% of hospitalized patients in withdrawal. It most commonly presents with the onset of delirium and significant autonomic hyperactivity, particularly tremor, tachycardia, and sometimes fever. Patients often develop visual hallucinations, which can be treated with neuroleptics.

Most acute episodes of withdrawal resolve within 2 weeks but can last 4 to 6 weeks. Rarely, mild symptoms of withdrawal can last months.

The present patient suffered from alcohol withdrawal syndrome, which, despite pharmacologic treatment, developed into delirium tremens. He required a lorazepam drip for 2 weeks; atenolol, 100 mg/d; and haloperidol (Haldol), 2 mg every 6 hours. He was eventually weaned off these medications by the third week. He also received nutritional supplementation. Although the patient had a mild coagulopathy secondary to alcohol use, he did not require any blood product support. The patient refused admission to an alcohol rehabilitation facility and was discharged home.

Clinical Pearls

1. Alcohol abusers who decrease alcohol intake to fewer than five drinks (60 g) per day have a lower rate of postoperative complications.

2. Alcohol withdrawal seizures can occur 8 hours after the last consumption and generally within the first 48 hours.

REFERENCES

1. Sullivan J, Sykoro K, Schneiderman J, et al: Assessment of alcohol withdrawal: The Revised Clinical Institute Withdrawal Assessment for Alcohol Scale (CIWA-Ar). Br J Addict 84:1353–1357, 1989.
2. American Psychiatric Association: Diagnostic and Statistical Manual of Mental Disorders, 4th ed. Washington, DC, American Psychiatric Association, 1994.
3. Lohr R: Treatment of alcohol withdrawal in hospitalized patients. Mayo Clin Proc 70:777–782, 1995.
4. Tonnensen H, Kehlet H: Preoperative alcoholism and postoperative morbidity. Br J Surg 86:869–874, 1999.
5. Chang PH, Steinberg MB: Alcohol withdrawal. Med Clin North Am 85:1191–1212, 2001.

PATIENT 49

A 73-year-old woman with a myocardial infarction after vascular surgery

A 73-year-old woman underwent a right femoral popliteal bypass for severe peripheral vascular disease. Her medical history is notable for a 25-year history of diabetes mellitus, hypertension, and hypothyroidism. She has no history of anginal symptoms. Her medications include lisinopril, metformin, and glyburide. On postoperative day 2, she has an increase in pulse associated with mild hypotension and tachypnea.

Physical Examination: Temperature 99°F, blood pressure 102/60. Neck: 2 cm jugular venous distention at 30°. Chest: rales of the lower lung fields. Heart: regular rhythm. Grade II/VI systolic murmur at the left sternal border. No rub or gallop. Abdomen: normal.

Laboratory Findings: WBC 7800/?μL, hematocrit 33%, platelets 178,000/μL. Electrolytes normal. BUN 31 mg/dL, creatinine 1.8 mg/dL. First creatine phosphokinase 405 mg/dL, CPK MB fraction 18%. Troponin 5.1 ng/dL. ECG: sinus tachycardia at a rate of 115, 2-mm ST depression in leads V1–V6 and inverted T waves leads I and aVL. Chest radiograph: mild pulmonary vascular congestion.

Question: What therapies are available to reduce the risk of postoperative myocardial ischemia and infarct?

Answer: Options include the β-blockers bisoprolol and atenolol, and the α$_2$-agonist mivazerol.

Discussion: Patients requiring vascular surgery for severe peripheral atherosclerosis have long been known to be at risk for postoperative myocardial ischemia and infarction. Several studies have examined what clinical characteristics put patients at high risk for perioperative cardiac events and what tests are valuable for identifying patients at risk. Studies also have evaluated therapies that can be used perioperatively to reduce the incidence of cardiac events in these patients.

The use of perioperative β-blockers has been studied and has been shown to be cardioprotective for patients who have coronary artery disease risk factors who are undergoing noncardiac surgeries. A study by Poldermans et al showed that the β-blocker bisoprolol decreased the rates of postoperative myocardial infarction and cardiac death in patients undergoing major vascular surgery for 2 years after the surgery. The patients all were identified as high cardiac risk based on the presence of one or more cardiac risk factors and a dobutamine echocardiogram positive for ischemia. Cardiac risk factors were defined as age >70 years, angina, previous myocardial infarction, compensated or prior congestive heart failure, current treatment for diabetes, current treatment for cardiac arrhythmias, and inability to perform most normal activities. The patients who received 5 to 10 mg of bisoprolol starting postoperatively and given daily over 2 years had a significant decrease in cardiac morbidity and mortality over that time period: The incidence of cardiac events during follow-up was 12% in the bisoprolol group versus 32% in the standard care group. A prior study by the same group showed that bisoprolol reduced cardiac events in the immediate postoperative period in the same class of patients.

Mangano et al conducted the first randomized, prospective trial on perioperative β-blockers. It showed that the use of perioperative atenolol in patients with risk factors for coronary artery disease undergoing noncardiac surgery was associated with a subsequent decrease in cardiac morbidity and mortality for 2 years postoperatively.

The perioperative atenolol protocol established by Mangano et al currently is used in various formats in several major centers. Patients are considered candidates for the protocol if they have two or more of the following cardiac risk factors: age >65, current smoking, diabetes requiring treatment, cholesterol >240 mg/dL, and hypertension. Patients also are candidates if they have known coronary artery disease. The protocol calls for atenolol in the immediate perioperative period. If the patient has no adverse effects (no wheezing, pulse >55 beats/min, systolic blood pressure >100 mmHg), the dose is repeated. The protocol also is repeated immediately postoperatively. The patient receives 50 to 100 mg of atenolol each day for 7 days or until discharge. If the patient receives nothing by mouth for a prolonged period postoperatively, the dose is 5 to 10 mg intravenously twice a day.

The α$_2$-agonist mivazerol also has been shown to reduce the risk of cardiac events in vascular surgery patients. Mivazerol may exert its cardioprotective effects by decreasing sympathetic activity and postganglionic norepinephrine availability, preventing catecholamine-induced increases in myocardial oxygen consumption. Further studies on mivazerol are forthcoming to validate its efficacy in the vascular population.

The present patient had not received perioperative β-blockers but was a candidate based on her risk factors of age, diabetes, and hypertension. Her postoperative myocardial infarction presented without any pain, a situation that occurs in 60% of postoperative cardiac events. The myocardial infarction was manifested by new congestive heart failure and a change in hemodynamic parameters. The patient received enoxaparin (Lovenox), aspirin, and β-blockers; her peak creatine phosphokinase was 859 mg/dL. A subsequent echocardiogram showed a significant anterolateral wall motion abnormality with a left ventricular ejection fraction of 30%. Perhaps perioperative β-blockers or mivazerol would have changed her outcome.

Clinical Pearls

1. Randomized trials of prophylactic nitroglycerin were too small to have the power to find any cardioprotective effects. A randomized trial of diltiazem also was too small.

2. It is not yet known if additional cardioprotective benefits could be achieved by adding perioperative mivazerol to perioperative β-blockers.

3. β-Blockers should be considered for all patients at high cardiac risk who require noncardiac surgery. Mivazerol may be considered for patients who cannot tolerate β-blockers.

REFERENCES

1. Mangano DT, Layug EL, Wallace A, et al: Effect of atenolol on mortality and cardiovascular morbidity after non-cardiac surgery. N Engl J Med 335:1713–1720, 1996.
2. Oliver MF, Goldman L, Julian DG, Hole I: Effect of mivazerol on perioperative cardiac complications during non-cardiac surgery in patients with coronary heart disease. Anesthesiology 91:951–961, 1999.
3. Fleisher LA, Eagle KA: Lowering cardiac risk in non-cardiac surgery. N Engl J Med 345:1677–1682, 2001.
4. Poldermans D, Boersma E, Bax JJ, et al: Bisoprolol reduces cardiac death and myocardial infarction in high-risk patients as long as 2 years after successful major vascular surgery. Eur Heart J 22:1353–1358, 2001.
5. Selzman CH, Miller SA, Zimmerman MA, Harken AH: The case for β-adrenergic blockade as prophylaxis against perioperative cardiovascular morbidity and mortality. Arch Surg 136:286–290, 2001.

PATIENT 50

A 69-year-old woman with a permanent cardiac pacemaker requiring lumbar laminectomy and fusion for spinal stenosis

A 69-year-old woman with a permanent cardiac pacemaker presents for lumbar laminectomy and fusion for spinal stenosis. She had a dual-chamber DDD pacer placed the previous year for third-degree heart block. At the time of surgery, she has a paced rate of 70 beats/min. Her cardiac review of systems is benign. Her pacer has a variable pacing rate depending on the rate of atrial contraction. It has a minimal ventricular pacing rate that is triggered if the atrial P wave rate is too low and a maximal ventricular pacing rate that is triggered if the P wave rate is higher than the programmed maximal ventricular rate (the pacer can return to atrioventricular synchrony by creating a Wenckebach block).

Physical Examination: Temperature 98°F, pulse 70, respirations 16, blood pressure 118/68. Chest: clear. Heart: paced rate, paradoxical S_2 owing to pacer-induced bundle-branch block. Grade I/VI systolic ejection murmur at the left sternal border.

Laboratory Findings: Electrolytes normal. CBC normal. ECG: rate 70, pacer spikes present with pacer-induced left bundle-branch block (see Figure).

Question: What is the major risk to pacemakers intraoperatively?

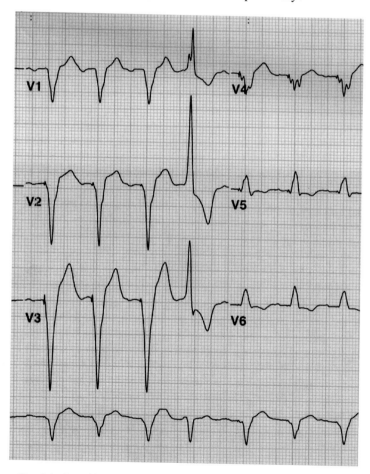

Paced rhythm with LBBB pattern. Pacer spikes visible in V_2 and V_3.

Answer: Use of cautery can intefere with pacer function.

Discussion: Newer pacemakers are pulse generators, which should not be electrically reset by surgical electrocautery. Older pacemakers can be electrically reset, however, during the use of cautery. Because of this possibility, the pacer probably should be interrogated postoperatively.

Electrocautery produces electromagnetic signals that can affect pacemakers in the following way: First, a pacer sensing a continuous burst of electromagnetic signals probably would sense it as noise and revert to an asynchronous pacing mode. Also, if the pacer senses more infrequent electromagnetic pulses, it may interpret them as intrinsic cardiac activity and inhibit pacing. If the electrocautery is sensed only in the atrial portion of a dual-chamber pacer, the atrial signal may be tracked to the ventricular channel, allowing the pacer to pace at its upper rate limit.

Pacemakers respond to magnets in a variety of ways. Most pacers respond to magnet placement by converting to an asynchronous mode in which all sensing functions are turned off, and the pulse generator fires at a predictable rate. Many new pacers have a program that can make magnet application ineffective. Some pacers respond to magnet application with only brief asynchronous pacing. Because the response to magnet application is variable depending on the pacer, it is important to obtain information from the pacer manufacturer when possible. Also, a magnet should not be placed routinely over a pacemaker generator during surgery. If the magnet is in place over a programmable pacer during the use of cautery, the pacer may become reprogrammed. In some pacers, the rate can revert to previously programmed parameters with the magnet still in place. The use of a magnet may be safe, however, in nonprogrammable pacers.

A variety of metabolic and acid-base abnormalities can increase the myocardial threshold for depolarization, potentially inhibiting myocardial capture of pacemaker impulses. Hypokalemia, hypercalcemia, hypomagnesemia, and severe acidosis or alkalosis all can cause loss of capture and should be corrected promptly.

Patients who have implantable cardioverter-defibrillators (ICDs) should have the device deactivated before surgery. If left on during surgery, an ICD could sense electrocautery as an arrhythmia and discharge in error. Some ICD models can respond by undersensing arrhythmias. To deactivate, a magnet can be placed over the ICD. The magnet prevents detection of dysrhythmias but does not affect pacing functions of the unit.

The present patient did not have her pacemaker interrogated before or after surgery. Cautery was used in short bursts, with ground plate away from the pulse generator. Her postoperative recovery was benign.

Management of Electrocautery in the Presence of a Pacemaker

1. Position the cautery grounding pad away from the pulse generator so that the generator is not in the path of cautery current flow.
2. Use cautery in short bursts.
3. Use the lowest possible current.
4. Do not use cautery over the pulse generator or along the lead path to the heart.
5. If pacer inhibition occurs, a magnet may be placed over the pulse generator. Most pacers respond by initiating asynchronous pacing.

Clinical Pearls

1. In the event that a pacer-dependent patient loses pacemaker function, noninvasive transthoracic pacing should be available in the operating room.

2. Because patients with ICDs often have significant ischemic heart disease and significant left ventricular dysfunction, they should be watched carefully in the intraoperative and postoperative periods for cardiac compromise.

3. For patients undergoing electroconvulsive therapy, the sensing mode should be changed to asynchronous pacing before the procedure because the seizure activity induced by electroconvulsive therapy could be sensed as intrinsic myocardial activity.

REFERENCES
1. Bourke ME: The patient with a pacemaker or related device. Can J Anaesth 43:R24–R32, 1996.
2. Rozner MA, Gursoy S, Monir G: Care of the patient with a pacemaker. In Stone DJ, Boddonoff DL, Leisure GS, et al (eds): Perioperative Care. St. Louis, Mosby, 1998, pp 53–67.
3. Sloan SB, Weitz HH: Postoperative arrhythmias and conduction disorders. Med Clin North Am 85:1171–1189, 2001.

PATIENT 51

A 72-year-old man with persistent confusion after coronary artery bypass graft surgery

A 72-year-old man underwent three-vessel coronary artery bypass graft surgery and mitral valve replacement. His past medical history was notable for hypertension and hyperlipidemia. His intraoperative course was without complication. Postoperatively, he was significantly confused. A month later, his confusion has cleared significantly, but it is noted by his family that his short-term memory is impaired significantly, and he no longer can do crossword puzzles or conduct his financial matters as he has in the past.

Physical Examination: Pulse 74, blood pressure 156/90. HEENT: normal. Chest: clear. Heart: regular rhythm. Mechanical S_1. No murmur. Well-healed midline sternotomy scar. Abdomen: benign.

Laboratory Findings: Electrolytes: normal. CBC: WBC 5400/μL, hematocrit 35%, platelets 193,000/μL. Total cholesterol 201 mg/dL, LDL 135 mg/L, HDL 40 mg/L.

Question: What are the clinical factors associated with neurologic compromise after cardiac surgery?

Answer: Some of the clinical factors associated with postoperative neurologic compromise in this setting include proximal aortic atherosclerosis, age > 70, diabetes, hypertension, and history of neurologic disease.

Discussion: It long has been known that the use of **cardiopulmonary bypass** during surgery is related to postoperative neurologic dysfunction. It has been difficult to evaluate the prevalence and types of postoperative neurologic dysfunction because clinical definitions, study designs, and timing of patient evaluations have varied significantly from study to study. The reported prevalence of stroke varies from 0.4% to 5.4%; the incidence of neuropsychologic dysfunction varies from 25% to 79%. One study showed subtle, residual change 6 months later, with most patients normalizing by 1 year. Two classes of problems have been identified. The first is the occurrence of a major event, such as coma, death, cerebrovascular accident, or transient ischemic attack. The second is the occurrence of a change in neuropsychologic functioning (sometimes referred to as *diffuse encephalopathy* or *global hypoperfusion syndrome*). A prospective observational study by Roach et al delineated type 1 and type 2 problems (see Table below). They found several independent predictors of type 1 and type 2 events that were statistically significant (Table at right). Proximal aortic atherosclerosis was the strongest independent predictor. This finding is consistent with the theory that most perioperative strokes are secondary to atherosclerotic emboli generated by surgical manipulation of the aorta. Other predictors, such as diabetes and hypertension, may reflect generalized atherosclerosis and abnormal au-

Predictors of Type 1 and Type 2
Neurologic Events

Type 1
  Age > 70
  History of pulmonary disease
  History of hypertension
  Moderate-to-severe proximal aortic
    atherosclerosis
  History of neurologic disease
  Diabetes mellitus
  History of unstable angina
Type 2
  Age > 70
  Excessive alcohol use
  Postoperative dysrhythmia
  History of coronary artery bypass graft
    surgery
  History of peripheral vascular disease
  History of pulmonary disease
  History of hypertension

toregulation. Advanced age is likely a marker for atherosclerosis and changes in autoregulation.

Some of the causes of stroke and neurologic dysfunction, such as particulate and air embolism, have decreased as techniques of cardiopulmonary bypass have improved. Using careful aortic cross-clamping, membrane oxygenators, arterial filters, and limited bypass time have been associated with decreased rates of embolism. Other problems, such as hyperviscosity caused by hypothermia, hypothermia-induced vasoconstriction, and end-organ hypoperfusion, still are sometimes an issue. A variety of medications have been used in an attempt to find one with neuroprotective effects; these include steroids, prostacyclines, barbiturates, calcium channel blockers, and *N*-methyl-d-asparate (NMDA). Nothing has yet been found consistently to be helpful. At this point, although risk factors for postoperative neurologic dysfunction have been delineated better, preventive and therapeutic techniques still need to be identified.

The present patient underwent neuropsychologic testing 8 months after surgery. He was found to have moderate memory impairment and deficits with spatial tasks and problem solving.

Type 1 and Type 2 Neurologic Events

Type 1
  Death due to stroke or hypoxic encephalopathy
  Nonfatal stroke
  Transient ischemic attack
  Coma or stupor by the time of discharge
Type 2
  New worsening of intellectual function
  Confusion
  Agitation
  Disorientation
  Memory deficit
  Seizure without evidence of focal injury

Clinical Pearls

1. In some studies, the most significant risk for postoperative ischemic injury has been a history of preoperative stroke.

2. The greatest predictors of risk for developing neuropsychologic deficits are advanced age and prolonged cardiopulmonary bypass.

3. A study using the antioxidant pegorgotein showed no reduction in postbypass neuropsychologic deficits.

4. Performance of combined carotid endarterectomy and coronary artery bypass graft surgery has an estimated 17% morbidity and mortality and should be performed only in patients whose neurologic and cardiac systems are unstable.

REFERENCES

1. Pugsley W, Klinger L, Paschalis C, et al: The impact of microemboli during cardiopulmonary bypass on neuropsychological functioning. Stroke 25:1393–1399, 1994.
2. Sotaniemi KA: Long-term neurologic outcome after cardiac operation. Ann Thorac Surg 1336–1339, 1995.
3. Mora CT, Henson MB, Weintraub WS, et al: The effect of temperature management during cardiopulmonary bypass on neurologic and neurophysiologic outcomes in patients undergoing coronary revascularization. J Thorac Cardiovasc Surg 112:514–522, 1996.
4. Roach GW, Kanchuger M, Mangano CM, et al: Adverse cerebral outcomes after coronary bypass surgery. N Engl J Med 335:1857–1863, 1996.
5. DiBenedetto DJ, Leisure GS, Tribble CG: Cardiopulmonary bypass. In Stone DJ, Bogdonoff DL, Leisure GS, et al (eds): Perioperative Care. St. Louis, Mosby, 1998, pp 609–622.
6. Butterworth J: A randomized blinded trial of the antioxidant pegorgotein: No reduction in neuropsychological deficits, inotropic drug support, or myocardial ischemia after coronary artery bypass surgery. J Cardiothorac Vasc Anesth 13:690–694, 1999.

PATIENT 52

A 58-year-old man with type 2 diabetes mellitus requiring urgent herniorrhaphy

A 58-year-old man with type 2 diabetes mellitus underwent surgery for an incarcerated inguinal hernia. He states that his fasting glucose is generally well controlled in the 100 to 140 mg/dL range. Postoperatively, his glucose is in the 240 to 300 mg/dL range. His usual medications are metformin, 1,000 mg twice a day, and glyburide, 10 mg once a day.

Physical Examination: Temperature 98.2°F, pulse 92, respirations 18, blood pressure 143/90. HEENT: bilateral early cataracts, fundi not well visualized, oropharynx clear. Lungs: bibasilar rales, which clear with cough. Cardiac: regular rhythm. No murmur, rub, or gallop. Abdomen: soft, hypoactive bowel sounds, surgical wound clean and moderately tender; nonfluctuant. Extremities: no edema or tenderness.

Laboratory Findings: WBC 10,900/μL, hematocrit 37.8%, platelets 304,000/μL. Serum sodium 136 mEq/L, potassium 4.0 mEq/L, chloride 97 mEq/L, bicarbonate 26 mEq/L, BUN 40 mg/dL, creatinine 1.7 mg/dL. Urine culture: no growth. Blood cultures: no growth. ECG: normal sinus rhythm with no ischemic changes.

Question: What causes postoperative worsening in diabetics?

Answer: Surgical stress causes increased secretion of glucagon, cortisol, and growth hormone, all of which induce hyperglycemia. Perioperative catecholamine surges also increase serum glucose levels.

Discussion: Because of changes in counter-regulatory hormones, insulin secretion, and insulin sensitivity, diabetics should be expected to have some degree of postoperative hyperglycemia. This situation is confounded by nutritional issues such as degree of enteral or parenteral feeding, degree of illness, and other factors such as concurrent infection, all of which are known to cause hyperglycemia. The degree to which any given patient will have postoperative hyperglycemia is difficult to predict.

Surgical stress results in the secretion of glucagon, growth hormone, cortisol, and catecholamines. Growth hormone, cortisol, and glucagon all enhance gluconeogenesis and glycogenolysis, resulting in hyperglycemia. Catecholamines cause increased insulin resistance and decreased insulin secretion, with an end result of hyperglycemia. Hyperglycemia generally lasts 3 to 5 days, at which time levels of catecholamines and hormones normalize.

Standard medication management for patients on oral agents consists of holding the oral agents approximately 1 day before surgery to avoid intraoperative and postoperative hypoglycemia, followed by use of an insulin sliding scale and frequent glucose checks intraoperatively and postoperatively. Although an insulin drip can be used, the degree of postoperative hyperglycemia does not generally require this in a patient with type 2 diabetes.

Preoperatively, oral agents are held according to their half-lives and mode of action (Table). Sulfonylureas generally are given last on the morning before surgery. For patients who take these agents twice a day and have less than optimal control, they can be given safely the night before surgery. If these agents are taken inadvertently on the morning of surgery, surgery does not need to be postponed, but careful attention should be paid to the patient's glucose levels. For patients using metformin, past recommendations have been to stop the medication 48 to 72 hours before surgery or before procedures requiring use of iodinated contrast material, to decrease the risk of postprocedure lactic acidosis. The risk of lactic acidosis now is believed to be low; current recommendations are for patients to continue the medication until the day before surgery, but the patients should receive adequate hydration. If there is postoperative worsening of renal function, the medication should be held. In the case of contrast material, metformin still is held 48 hours preprocedure if possible. The thiazolidinediones can be held on the morning of surgery. Repaglinide also can be held the morning of surgery; this agent is used with meals and has a half-life of only 30 minutes. α-Glucosidase inhibitors also are used only with meals and can be held starting the morning of surgery. These agents prevent glucose absorption at the intestinal brush border and so are useful only in conjunction with oral intake.

Oral agents can be resumed after surgery when patients begin oral intake. Initially, oral intake postoperatively often is only a fraction of a patient's usual degree of intake. In this case, consider starting oral agents at half the usual dose. If the patient is taking more than one oral agent, the physician should consider starting them one at a time, observing the glucose response.

For type 2 diabetics who require insulin, the basic regimen for the day of surgery is for the patient to receive one third to one half of the usual morning insulin dose but no regular insulin. The patient should concurrently receive intravenous fluids containing dextrose and regular insulin according

Oral Agents

Class	Mechanism of Action	Perioperative Management
Sulfonylureas	Stimulates insulin secretion from the pancreas	Hold 24 hours preoperatively. Restart when patient is eating
Biguanides (metformin)	Augments peripheral glucose uptake, sensitizes peripheral tissues to insulin. Inhibits gluconeogenesis	Hold 24 hours preoperatively; 48 hours if contrast to be used. Restart postoperatively when eating and after renal function checked
Thiazolidinediones	Improves peripheral glucose uptake, inhibits hepatic gluconeogenesis	Hold on the morning of surgery. Resume when patient eating
α-Glucosidase inhibitors	Prevents glucose absorption at the intestinal brush border.	Hold on the morning of surgery. Resume when patient is eating
Meglitinides	Stimulates insulin secretion from the pancreas	Hold on the morning of surgery. Resume when patient is eating

to a sliding scale. The patient also should receive half of the usual evening NPH. The insulin can be titrated back to the patient's usual doses as oral intake increases postoperatively.

The present patient had postoperative worsening of diabetes for 3 days. The elevations were not unexpected, but to ensure no confounding processes such as infection or ischemia, he was evaluated with an ECG, troponin level, urine culture, blood culture, and physical examination. The patient was not found to have any secondary processes. Because his glucose was high, when he began eating, both of his oral agents were resumed at the same time. He tolerated this well, and his serum glucose was in the 140 to 170 mg/dL range when he was discharged on postoperative day 5.

Clinical Pearls

1. The physician should consider starting the combination oral agent Glucovance, which consists of glyburide and metformin, as its separate components postoperatively if the patient is not eating well, to help avoid postoperative hypoglycemia.

2. The chemotaxis and phagocytosis of WBCs is impaired above a blood glucose level of 220 mg/dL; the major postoperative goal for glycemic control is to keep blood glucose below that level.

3. Ringer's lactate intravenous solution can worsen hyperglycemia because the lactate is metabolized to glucose by the liver. Ringer's lactate, 1 L, produces 22 g of glucose when metabolized.

REFERENCES

1. Hirsch IB, McGill JB, Cryer PE, White PF: Perioperative management of surgical patients with diabetes mellitus. Anesthesiology 74:346–359, 1991.
2. Schiff RL, Emanuele MA: The surgical patient with diabetes mellitus. J Gen Intern Med 10:154–161, 1995.
3. Jacober SJ, Sowers JR: An update on perioperative management of diabetes. Arch Intern Med 159:2405–2411, 1999.
4. McAnulty GR, Robertshaw HJ, Hall GM: Anaesthetic management of patients with diabetes mellitus. Br J Anaesth 85:80–90, 2000.

PATIENT 53

A 36-year-old man with type 1 diabetes mellitus and an acute abdomen

A 36-year-old man with type 1 diabetes mellitus is admitted for evaluation of an acute abdomen. He has a 3-day history of worsening upper and lower right-sided abdominal pain, decreasing appetite, and chills. His diabetes is complicated by mild retinopathy and neuropathy. He also has a history of hypertension. His medications are lisinopril; gabapentin (Neurontin); and an insulin regimen consisting of NPH, 24 U a.m. and 16 U p.m., and Regular, 10 U a.m. and 6 U p.m. He is scheduled for a laparotomy for suspected appendicitis.

Physical Examination: Temperature 100.7°F, pulse 128, respirations 20, blood pressure 148/74. Oxygen saturation 97% room air. General appearance: uncomfortable-appearing young man. Chest: clear. Heart: tachycardia. Normal S_1 and S_2, no murmur. Abdomen: hypoactive bowel sounds, guarding and pain on palpation of the right upper quadrant and right midabdomen. Significant rebound tenderness. No masses. Extremities: no edema. Skin: no jaundice. Neurologic: deep tendon reflexes 2+ and equal throughout. Strength intact. Sensation decreased to light touch and pinprick of the bilateral feet just above the ankles.

Laboratory Findings: WBC 18,600/μL, 18% bands, 70% polymorphonuclear neutrophils, 12% lymphocytes. Hematocrit 39.2%, platelets 287,000/μL. Sodium 132 mEq/L, potassium 3.8 mEq/L, chloride 94 mEq/L, bicarbonate 20 mEq/L, BUN 27 mg/dL, creatinine 1.3 mg/dL, glucose 431 mg/dL. β-hydroxybutyrate 3.6 mmol/L. Lactate 4.1, total bilirubin 1.6 mg/dL. AST, ALT, alkaline phosphatase, amylase, and lipase: all normal. Anion gap: 18.

Question: What are the main postoperative complications in type 1 diabetics?

Answer: In addition to hyperglycemia, type 1 diabetics can have poor wound healing, postoperative cardiac ischemia, and possible cardiorespiratory arrest if autonomic dysfunction is present.

Discussion: A primary perioperative issue for patients with type 1 diabetes is the maintenance of an adequate degree of insulin therapy. Glucose must be provided to avoid initiation of protein catabolism, lipolysis, and ketogenesis.

Glucose should be given for metabolic needs: Intravenous fluids containing 5% dextrose and delivered at 100 mL/h provides 5 g of glucose per hour, or 120 g in 24 hours. Most daily metabolic requirements are in the range of 120 to 240 g/d. Conversely, the pancreas usually produces 0.5 to 1.0 U of insulin per hour, which can metabolize 8.4 g of glucose per hour. The stress of surgery can increase insulin requirements twofold to threefold. In general, an insulin drip of 1.0 to 2.0 U/h can maintain blood glucose levels between 100 and 200 mg/dL for most diabetics perioperatively. This approach is most useful for all type 1 diabetics and poorly controlled type 2 diabetics undergoing major surgery. For well-controlled type 1 diabetics, the most common insulin regimen consists of one half to one third of the morning NPH or Lente, followed by sliding scale Regular Insulin. If the patient is eating the evening of surgery, one half of the usual NPH can be given again, with continued sliding scale Regular Insulin every 6 hours in conjunction with glucose monitoring. If the patient is eating full meals, full-dose NPH or Lente can be given. If intravenous fluids need to be restricted, glucose can be given as 20% or 50% solution. Lactated Ringer's solution should not be used for diabetics because the lactate undergoes rapid metabolism to glucose. Insulin can never be held perioperatively in type 1 diabetics, even when they have no oral intake. Initiation of lipolysis, ketogenesis, and protein catabolism would occur.

Patients with diabetic ketoacidosis always present in a state of volume depletion and require vigorous intravenous volume repletion and aggressive correction of electrolyte abnormalities. Patients with diabetic ketoacidosis routinely should be considered to require significant potassium repletion. When the serum potassium is <4.0 mEq/L, potassium chloride should be added to all intravenous fluids. (As the patient's acidosis is corrected, potassium is driven intracellularly, decreasing serum potassium levels.)

Common perioperative issues for diabetics include problems with wound healing, an increased risk of postoperative ischemia, complications resulting from renal dysfunction, and complications resulting from autonomic neuropathy. Poor WBC functioning occurs in diabetics when glucose is >220 mg/dL and possibly >200 mg/dL; this can contribute to increased risk of wound infection and abscess formation. Wound healing can be delayed because hyperglycemia decreases collagen synthesis. Diabetics have a higher risk of perioperative infection than nondiabetics, and 20% of all perioperative deaths in diabetics are secondary to infection.

The most common cause of perioperative death in diabetics is cardiac disease. Diabetes has been found to be an independent predictor of cardiac events in vascular surgery and for increased mortality in cardiac surgery; this is in keeping with the fact that diabetics have a higher risk of coronary artery disease. Diabetics with autonomic insufficiency have a higher risk of sudden cardiac and respiratory arrest perioperatively. Autonomic dysfunction also can cause decreased bladder tone, with an increased risk of postoperative urinary retention and an increased incidence of orthostatic hypotension, which can cause problems with postoperative ambulation. Gastroparesis also can be a perioperative problem for diabetics. Delayed gastric emptying can result in full or partially full gastric contents at the time of anesthetic induction, increasing the risk of aspiration.

Other perioperative issues in diabetics include renal dysfunction and metabolic abnormalities. Renal function should be monitored, and anesthetic agents with the least nephrogenic toxicity should be chosen. Electrolytes, particularly potassium, should be followed. Patients taking angiotensin-converting enzyme inhibitors are often hyperkalemic, whereas patients with diabetic ketoacidosis are generally hypokalemic.

The present patient was found to have appendicitis with abscess formation. He had mild ketoacidosis; most of his anion gap was due to a lactic acidosis. He received vigorous hydration and 10 U of insulin, followed by an insulin drip of 2 U/h. He went to surgery after he had received the insulin bolus and initiation of the insulin drip. His plasma glucose was 290 mg/dL when surgery started. His glucose remained at 240–300 mg/dl postoperatively on the insulin drip. On the first postoperative day, his insulin drip was titrated down when his glucose level improved further. On the second postoperative day, the patient's usual regimen was restarted and titrated to keep his glucose in the range of 100 to 200 mg/dL.

Clinical Pearls

1. Insulin requirements for patients receiving total parenteral nutrition are usually higher than they were when the patients were eating preoperatively. This is secondary to gastrointestinal factors such as glucose-lowering peptides, which affect enteral delivery of food.

2. Patients receiving total parenteral nutrition should have insulin added directly to the total parenteral nutrition and additional intermediate-acting and short-acting insulin subcutaneously titrated to the target plasma glucose range.

3. Rapid-acting insulin should be changed to Regular Insulin because the timing of the patient's hospital meal may not be immediately after his or her injection.

4. Long-acting insulin (i.e., Ultralente or insulin glargine) does not offer flexibility for an inpatient with unpredictable oral intake. The physician should consider changing the patient to a combination of intermediate-acting and short-acting insulin.

REFERENCES

1. Hirsch IB, McGill JB, Cryer PE, White PF: Perioperative management of surgical patients with diabetes mellitus. Anesthesiology 74:346–359, 1991.
2. McGlynn TJ, Simons RJ: Endocrine disorders. In Gross RJ, Caputo GM (eds): Medical Consultation. Baltimore, Williams & Wilkins, 1998, pp 329–333.
3. Jacober SJ, Sowers JR: An update on perioperative management of diabetes. Arch Intern Med 159:2405–2411, 1999.
4. McAnulty GR, Robertshaw HJ, Hall GM: Anaesthetic management of diabetes with diabetes mellitus. Br J Anesth 85:80–90, 2000.
5. Hoogwerf BJ: Postoperative management of the diabetic patient. Med Clin North Am 85:1213–1228, 2001.

PATIENT 54

A 61-year-old woman on multiple medications presenting
for preoperative evaluation

A 61-year-old woman on multiple medications is being evaluated preoperatively before undergoing a radical mastectomy. Her past medical history is notable for hyperlipidemia, osteoporosis, hypothyroidism, hypertension, a history of paroxysmal atrial fibrillation, and peripheral vascular disease. Her medications include atorvastatin, raloxifene (Evista), levothyroxine, lisinopril, hydrochlorothiazide, amiodarone, aspirin, and cilostazol (Pletal).

Physical Examination: Temperature 98.2°F, pulse 72, blood pressure 154/80. Funduscopic examination: mild arteriolar narrowing and occasional arteriovenous nicking. Optic disks normal. Chest: clear. Cardiac: regular rate and rhythm. Grade II/VI systolic ejection murmur at the lower left sternal border. Abdomen: benign. Extremities: left femoral bruit present. Lower extremities with no hair present. Dorsalis pedis and posterior tibial pulses not palpable. Mild dependent rubor present. Feet cool to the touch. No edema.

Laboratory Findings: Sodium 135 mEq/dL, potassium 3.5 mEq/dL, chloride 97 mEq/dL, bicarbonate 27 mEq/dL, BUN 27 mg/dL, creatinine 1.3 mg/dL. CBC: normal.

Question: How should medications be managed perioperatively?

Answer: The antiplatelet agents aspirin and cilostazol should be stopped, and the raloxifene should be stopped as well.

Discussion: Medical consultants often are asked to manage a wide variety of medications perioperatively, but there is little literature available to guide management. Prospective studies are almost nonexistent, and the available retrospective studies of medications often involve small numbers of patients. Decisions sometimes are made based on anecdotal evidence or theoretical issues. Although older standards of care involved stopping medications for a variable time preoperatively, most medicines now are continued perioperatively, including the day of surgery.

Antihypertensive medications are continued perioperatively, including the day of surgery. The exception to this is hydrochlorothiazide, which some physicians hold on the day of surgery to help avoid intravascular volume depletion at the time of induction of anesthesia. The volume depletion can accentuate anesthesia-induced hypotension. One also can consider holding angiotensin-converting enzyme inhibitors on the morning of surgery because there are reports that these agents can cause hypotension. Antianginal medications should be continued on the day of surgery. Nitrate patches can be converted to an oral form because transdermal delivery in the operating room when the patient may be cold is unpredictable. Some anesthesiologists continue the transdermal form but are prepared to add intravenous nitrates should frank ischemia develop. β-Blockers have been especially impressive in decreasing perioperative cardiac morbidity and mortality and are discussed elsewhere in this book. Oral hypoglycemics, another commonly used class of medication, also are discussed elsewhere.

The present patient was on a wide variety of medications. She was taking raloxifene (Evista), which is a selective estrogen receptor modulator that has been found to be a useful osteoporosis medication because of it estrogen-like effects on bone. Similar to tamoxifen, however, raloxifene increases the risk of venous thromboembolism. The risk is greatest in the first 4 months of therapy. Even after the first 4 months, if a patient requires surgery, the medication should be stopped at least 72 hours preoperatively and resumed only when the patient is fully mobile.

For patients who are on bisphosphonate medication for osteoporosis therapy, although there are no specific contraindications or medication interactions, they are difficult to take properly and are best held in acutely ill patients. (The patient must take the medication on an empty stomach with a full glass of water and must remain upright for 30 minutes.)

If a patient is on estrogen replacement therapy, this too has been found to have increased risk of postoperative venous thromboembolism. It is unclear how long in advance of surgery the estrogen should be stopped; one report suggested 1 month. Birth control pills should be held for 1 month preoperatively, although the risks and benefits of accidental pregnancy and alternate methods of birth control should be discussed with the patient.

The present patient also was taking lisinopril and hydrochlorothiazide. As mentioned earlier, one could hold both of these medications the morning of surgery to avoid hypotension. Other blood pressure medications usually are given routinely on the morning of surgery. Because the present patient likely had coronary artery disease given her significant peripheral vascular disease, she would have benefited from the ischemic protection offered by perioperative β-blockers, which would lend the added benefit of controlling her hypertension.

For lower extremity claudication, the present patient was taking cilostazol (Pletal), which is a phosphodiesterase inhibitor. It causes dilation of vascular beds and is an antiplatelet agent. Its action on platelets is reversible, and the half-life is approximately 12 hours; it should be discontinued 3 days preoperatively. The other commonly used antiplatelet agents, ticlopidine (Ticlid) and clopidogrel (Plavix), are thienopyridines, which irreversibly inhibit adenosine diphosphate–induced platelet aggregation but which do not have any direct effects on arachidonic acid metabolism. These medications should be stopped 7 days preoperatively when possible. Dipyridamole has antiplatelet and vasodilator activities; the main mechanism of action is not fully known. It has reversible action on platelets and a half-life of 10 hours; it should be stopped 2 to 3 days preoperatively. Aspirin impedes platelet activity by irreversibly inhibiting platelet cyclooxygenase. The general standard of care is to discontinue aspirin 7 to 10 days preoperatively because the circulating platelet pool is replaced every 7 to 10 days. Although it has been known to increase the amount of bleeding intraoperatively, there is no evidence for a resultant significant increase in morbidity and mortality. The only exception would be neurosurgeries and vascular surgeries, in which excessive bleeding can increase morbidity significantly. Other nonsteroidal agents reversibly inhibit platelet cyclooxygenase and can be held 3 days preoperatively. The newer nonsteroidal anti-inflammatory drugs (cyclooxygenase-2 inhibitors) are thought to have less effect on platelet function than the older agents. Their half-life is fairly short (17 hours for rofecoxib and 11 hours for celecoxib), and they should be stopped 4 to 5 days preoperatively.

The use of amiodarone is increasingly common, especially in the treatment of atrial fibrillation. It has an extremely long half-life (20 days, with an increase to 47 days in patients >65 years old), so holding it in the immediate perioperative period serves no clinical purpose. It has been associated with rare reports of postoperative adult respiratory distress syndrome, the mechanism of which is unclear. Amiodarone is available in an intravenous form if needed for serious arrhythmias. As with amiodarone, other antiarrhythmics should be continued perioperatively. The proarrhythmic effects of antiarrhythmics are accentuated by conditions such as hypokalemia, hypomagnesemia, and hypocalcemia. Such electrolyte and divalent abnormalities should be monitored and corrected perioperatively.

Digoxin can be given the morning of surgery, but the level should be checked preoperatively. Common conditions such as hypoxia, acidosis, hypokalemia, and increased catecholamines can increase digoxin toxicity and should be treated appropriately.

Medications used to treat dyslipidemias should be stopped the day before surgery. Drugs that bind bile acids (cholestyramine and colestipol) may decrease bioavailability of other oral medications, which may affect the treatment of hospitalized patients. The hydroxymethylglutaryl coezyme A (HMG-CoA) derivatives and niacin can cause severe myopathy, which can lead to rhabdomyolysis. They also may provoke muscle injury that occurs perioperatively.

The patient also was taking levothyroxine for hypothyroidism. This medication has a long half-life of approximately 7 days. It can be taken perioperatively including the morning of surgery because it is not associated with any adverse interactions with anesthetics, but if one or two doses are missed, it should not have any adverse clinical effect.

The present patient did not stop raloxifene preoperatively and developed a deep venous thrombosis in the postoperative period. It was thought that the raloxifene contributed to her deep venous thrombosis. She had stopped aspirin and cilostazol 1 week before the surgery and restarted them on postoperative day 1. The patient took all of her other medications perioperatively, including the day of surgery.

Clinical Pearls

1. Although most medications are safe to continue perioperatively, it is wise to hold any unnecessary medications on the day of surgery.

2. Preoperative medication levels should be checked when appropriate (digoxin, theophylline, phenytoin).

3. Herbal medications should be held 1 to 2 weeks preoperatively. Several of these agents have been found to have adverse interactions with anesthetic medications and to have antiplatelet activity.

REFERENCES

1. Smith MS, Muir H, Hall R: Perioperative management of drug therapy, clinical considerations. Drugs 51:238–259, 1996.
2. Kroenke K, Gooby-Toedt D, Jackson JL: Chronic medications in the perioperative period. South Med J 91:358–364, 1998.
3. Haynes B, Dowsett M: Clinical pharmacology of selective estrogen receptor modulators. Drugs Aging 14:323–336, 1999.
4. Grady D, Wenger NK, Herrington D, et al: Postmenopausal hormone therapy increases risk for venous thromboembolic disease. The Heart and Estrogen/progestin Replacement Study. Ann Intern Med 132:689–696, 2000.
5. Spell NO: Stopping and restarting medications in the perioperative period. Med Clin North Am 85:1117–1128, 2001.

PATIENT 55

An 86-year old woman requiring repair of a hip fracture

An 86-year-old resident of a nursing home tripped on another resident's walker and sustained an intertrochanteric hip fracture when she fell. Her past medical history is notable for osteoporosis, depression, hypertension, and hyperlipidemia. Her medications are Fosamax, Paxil, Norvasc, and Lipitor, as well as calcium carbonate.

Physical Examination: Blood pressure 170/96; pulse 110; respirations 16; temperature 99.6°F. Chest: clear. Cardiac: regular rate and rhythm, normal S1 and S2; grade 2/6 systolic murmur at the left sternal border. Abdomen: benign. Extremities: left leg shortened and externally rotated.

Laboratory Findings: WBC 10,000/µL, HCT 32%, platelets 180,000 cells/µL. Electrolytes normal. EKG: sinus tachycardia at a rate of 106; Q waves in leads II, III, and AVL; no significant ST or T wave changes. Hip x-ray: displaced left intertrochanteric fracture.

Question: What type of complications is this patient at risk for?

Answer: The most common complications in this setting are postoperative confusion, delirium, and poor functional recovery.

Discussion: As the population has aged, the occurrence of hip fractures has risen precipitously, as has the associated cost. In 1990, the number of reported hip fractures in the United States was 281,000, with an associated cost of greater than 8 billion dollars. The number of hip fractures is expected to double by the year 2040.

Just as preventive health care is critical to curbing the problem of hip fractures in the geriatric population, proactive medical care in the perioperative period is also critical. Problems common to the geriatric hip-fracture patient include malnutrition, urinary retention after removal of indwelling urinary catheters, delirium, and poor postoperative functional recovery. In addition, the type of hip fracture itself can influence the type of complications as well as the outcome.

Intertrochanteric fractures involve the cancellous bone between the greater and lesser trochanters and are extracapsular. They are most common in elderly patients and have a female to male ratio of approximately 5:1. There is very good vascular supply to the area because of the cancellous bone and because of the large amount of surrounding musculature; thus, postoperative avascular necrosis is uncommon. Although orthopedists use a more complex classification system, for the purposes of emergency medicine and medical consultation, intertrochanteric fractures can be classified as **stable** (no displacement between the femoral shaft and neck) and **unstable** (multiple fracture lines or comminution with associated displacement). Most of these fractures are due to direct trauma such as a fall.

The other two basic types of hip fracture are intracapsular and subtrochanteric. *Intracapsular fractures* (also called femoral neck fractures) can have a varying amount of displacement, from none to marked. In nondisplaced femoral neck fractures, since there is little interruption of bleed supply to the femoral head and good bony contact between the fracture surfaces, the required operation is small, involving only application of cannulated screws. A severely displaced femoral neck fracture bleeds more, often requires transfusion, and is repaired with hemiarthroplasty. There is a much higher risk of thromboembolism with this procedure, requiring appropriate postoperative anticoagulation.

Subtrochanteric fractures are proximal femur fractures. These, too, can be associated with significant bleeding requiring transfusion. Repairs involve either the placement of an intramedullary device or horizontal compression screws with a long side plate.

Up to 20% of patients admitted to the hospital with hip fracture are malnourished. Studies have shown that patients who received **protein supplementation** had shorter lengths of stay and achieved independent mobility faster than those who did not. The standard of care in geriatric patients should include measurement of nutritional status, with correction of deficiencies, especially protein.

Indwelling urinary catheters are used for a variable period postoperatively in hip-fracture patients. Some studies have shown that removal of the catheters within the first 24 hours postoperatively decreases both the rate of urinary tract infection and postoperative urinary retention. When possible, practitioners should attempt to remove catheters within 24 hours postoperatively and utilize intermittent straight catheterization.

The reported rate of **delirium** after repair of the fracture varies widely: rates as low as 9.5% and as high as 61% have been reported. Because of interference with participation in postoperative physical therapy, delirium can affect the eventual functional outcome and increase the risk of nursing home placement. A study by Brauer et al revealed that there is often not a clearly definable cause for postoperative delirium in hip fracture patients. Although it is important to rule out common causes of delirium (such as infectious, metabolic, endocrinologic, cardiopulmonary), it is likely multifactorial and may involve iatrogenic conditions related to the surgery, such as the effects of anesthesia and pain medications. Provide environmental cueing, behavioral redirection, and pharmacologic therapy for agitation and severe confusion.

It has been reported that the delay of surgical repair beyond 24 hours after injury increased morbidity and worsened long-term functional recovery. This is generally true, although patients sometimes have medical conditions which require postponing surgery for longer than 24 hours to achieve perioperative stabilization. Hospital mortality rates of hip-fracture patients have been reported as approximately 5%, with post-discharge increases to 13% at 3 months and 24% at 12 months after fracture. In addition, one study showed that only 50% of patients could walk unaided 1 year after fracture. Further studies are needed to better understand the high rates of morbidity and mortality associated with hip fracture and how to prevent them.

The present patient tolerated her surgery, but experienced delirium postoperatively for 3 days. She was treated with risperidone, and her mental status returned to baseline after 9 days. However, the delirium caused her postoperative physical therapy to be significantly delayed. One month after the fracture she still had not reached her preoperative functional baseline. Her age and history of hypertension, as well as the Q waves seen on EKG, indicated at least mild risk for a perioperative cardiac event. Since myocardial infarction in the postoperative period can present as confusion or delirium, she was also evaluated for an MI (the work-up was negative).

Clinical Pearls

1. Patients who have experienced hip fractures are at higher risk for subsequent falls.

2. Providing lower extremity exercise, balance training, and evaluating patients' individual risk factors for falls may help reduce subsequent falls and fractures in this population.

3. Many patients admitted for hip fractures have never had assessment or therapy for osteoporosis. These patients should receive outpatient osteoporosis evaluation and therapy after recovery from their fractures.

REFERENCES

1. Morrison RS, Chassin MR, Siu AL: The medical consultant's role in caring for patients with hip fracture. Ann Int Med 128: 1010–1020, 1998.
2. Brauer C, Morrison RS, Silberzweig SB, Siu AL: The cause of delirium in patients with hip fracture. Arch Int Med. 160: 1856–1860, 2000.
3. Lichtblau S: Hip fracture: Surgical decisions that affect medical management. Geriatrics 55: 50–56, 2000.
4. Huddleston JM, Whitford KJ: Medical care of elderly patients with hip fractures. Mayo Clin Proc 76: 295–298, 2001.

PATIENT 56

A 47-year-old woman with hypothyroidism, dyspnea, and a postoperative oxygen requirement

A 47-year-old, morbidly obese woman underwent a vertical banded gastroplasty under general anesthesia. Her past medical history was notable for hypothyroidism, sleep apena, and hypertension. One day after surgery, she developed progressive shortness of breath and was noted to have an oxygen saturation of 82%. She denied any pleuritic chest pain, anginal chest pain, orthopnea, cough, or sputum production. Her oxygen saturation transiently improved to 89% with deep inspiration.

Physical Exam: O_2 saturation 82% on room air, 93% on 2L O_2, temperature 98.8°F, pulse 68, respirations 20, blood pressure 122/66. HEENT: normal. Chest: shallow respirations, but clear to auscultation throughout. Cardiac: regular rate and rhythm, without murmurs or gallops. Extremities: normal.

Laboratory Findings: Hct 34.1%. Chemistries: normal. ECG: normal. Chest radiograph: normal. Ventilation perfusion scan: normal. Thyroid-stimulating hormone: 56.

Question: What is the most likely cause of the patient's shortness of breath?

Diagnosis: Postoperative respiratory muscle weakening from hypothyroidism

Discussion: Although mildly hypothyroid patients can undergo surgery without clinically significant side effects, patients with significant hypothyroidism are at risk for a wide range of intraoperative and postoperative problems. The pulmonary complications include pleural effusions, decreased hypoxic ventilatory drive with carbon dioxide retention, respiratory muscle weakness, and respiratory failure. There may be preoperative respiratory muscle weakness, which can worsen postoperatively. The combination of respiratory muscle weakness, narcotics, hypothermia, and miscellaneous postoperative pulmonary complications such as pneumonia can together cause **postoperative hypoxemia.** In the present case, the clinical scenario was consistent with respiratory muscle weakness and decreased hypoxic drive.

Other organ systems can also be affected postoperatively. Hypothyroid patients can develop SIADH, delayed gastric emptying, and ileus. Side effects to medications can be exacerbated by decreased drug metabolism, and patients can be profoundly sensitive to narcotics. Cardiovascular complications include severe hypotension, bradycardia, decreased cardiac output, conduction abnormalities, and cardiac arrest. Patients are also more sensitive to the effects of narcotics and anesthetic agents.

Elective surgery should be postponed until hypothyroidism can be corrected or at least improved into the realm of mild signs and symptoms. If surgery must occur, use glucocorticoids in stress doses, because adrenal insufficiency may coexist with the hypothyroidism. If possible, emergency surgery should be delayed for 48 hours after initiation of levothyroxine to allow time for the onset of thyroid hormone activity. A large dose of levothyroxine (300 mcg) by slow intravenous infusion is given only in the clinical setting of impending or overt myxedema coma, severe hypothermia, or infection. Patients who are not as severely affected can receive 200 mcg per day by slow IV infusion, followed by 1.7 mcg/kg/day. Employ continuous ECG monitoring for atrial or ventricular dysrhythmias. Patients who are elderly or who have a history of coronary artery disease are at risk of acute ischemia or infarction during initiation of thyroid hormone replacement; they should receive low initial doses at 25–50 mcg per day. This can be titrated up by 25–50 mcg/day every 2–4 weeks to a total of 1.7 mcg/kg/day.

The present patient was treated with oxygen at 3 L/min per nasal cannula. She received intravenous thyroxine in a dose of 200 mcg initially, followed by 300 mcg po daily. Her shortness of breath and hypoxemia were resolved by the seventh postoperative day. In retrospect, the patient admitted to significant preoperative fatigue, which she had attributed to her sleep apnea; worsening of her usual constipation; and a 40-pound weight gain over 6 months indicating that she had significant preoperative hypothyroidism.

Clinical Pearls

1. Overt hypothyroidism can cause significant intraoperative and postoperative pulmonary complications.

2 For severe symptoms, treat with 300 mcg levothyroxine intravenously per day.

3. Hold urgent surgery for 48 hours if possible to allow for onset of action of levothyroxine.

REFERENCES

1. Wilson WR, Bedell GN: The pulmonary abnormalities in myxedema. J Clin Invest 39:42–55, 1960.
2. Zwillich WC, Pierson DJ, Hofeldt FD, et al: Ventilatory control in myxedema an hypothyroidism. New Engl J Med 292:662–665, 1975.
3. Murkin JM: Anesthesia and hypothyroidism: A review of thyroxine physiology, pharmacology, and anesthetic complications. Anesth Anal 61:371–383, 1982.
4. Weinberg AD, Brennan MD, Gorman CA, et al: Outcome of anesthesia and surgery in hypothyroid patients. Arch Int Med 143:893–897, 1983.
5. Boulanger BR, Gann DS: Management of the trauma victim with pre-existing endocrine disease. Crit Care Clin 10:537–554, 1994.
6. Ayala AR, Danese MD, Ladenson PW: When to treat mild hypothyroidism. Endocrinol Metab Clin North Am 29:399–415, 2000.

PATIENT 57

A 77-year-old man with a postoperative stroke

A 77-year-old man undergoes repair of a fracture that he sustained during a fall on the ice. His past medical history is notable for hypertension and type 2 diabetes mellitus. He tolerates the surgical procedure without any apparent problem. Several hours after awakening, however, he develops a left-sided facial droop with left arm weakness and numbness.

Physical Examination: Temperature 99.8°F, pulse 88, respirations 18, blood pressure 174/96. Lungs: clear. Heart: normal S_1 and S_2. No murmurs, rubs, or gallops. Abdomen: benign. Neurologic: dysarthria, left facial droop, deviation of the tongue to the left, left homonymous hemianopsia, significant left upper and lower extremity weakness of the flexors and extensors. Sensation significantly decreased to pinprick and light touch. Deep tendon reflexes 3+ on the left. Positive left Babinski reflex.

Laboratory Findings: WBC 8,100/μL, hematocrit 33%, platelets 410,000/μL. Electrolytes, BUN, and creatinine all normal. Glucose 161 mg/dL. Head CT scan: hypodense area of the right parietal lobe, consistent with early findings of a stroke. ECG: normal sinus rhythm with no acute changes.

Question: What are the risk factors for perioperative stroke?

Answer: For general surgery patients, risks for perioperative stroke include atrial fibrillation, advanced age, hypertension, atherosclerosis, and intraoperative hypotension.

Discussion: The reported incidence of stroke after general surgery ranges from 0.08% to 2.9%. Although perioperative stroke is associated most commonly with vascular surgery, it is common in cardiac and neurologic procedures. Common causative factors are intraoperative hypotension and atrial fibrillation; other factors include carotid artery stenosis, post–carotid surgery thromboembolism, cerebral fat embolism, cardioembolic infarct after cardiac surgery, perioperative myocardial infarction with thromboembolism, septic emboli, and postoperative hypercoagulability. In general surgery, associated factors for perioperative stroke are atrial fibrillation, advanced age, atherosclerosis, and hypertension. In multiple studies of carotid endarterectomy patients, hypertension was found to be a significant risk factor.

A case-controlled study by Limburg et al[2] found three major independent risk factors for stroke after general surgery: (1) previous cerebrovascular disease, (2) chronic obstructive pulmonary disease, and (3) the presence of peripheral vascular disease. A minor predictor was higher blood pressure at the time of admission. Hypotension was not found to be a relevant factor. This was the first study in which chronic obstructive pulmonary disease was found to be a statistically significant factor.

Cardiac surgery has long been known to have an increased risk of intraoperative stroke. Multiple factors have been implicated, including aortic atherosclerosis at the site of clamping, microembolization of polyvinyl tubing and silicone, air embolism, cardiac dysrhythmia, hypotension, and length of cardiopulmonary bypass time.

Perioperative strokes has been characterized as occurring within two time frames: early (within 5 days of surgery) and late (between 5 days and 2 years after surgery). The occurrence of intraoperative strokes implies mechanisms such as hypoperfusion. The occurrence of this type of strokes varies widely from study to study, ranging from 17%–70%. This wide range likely is related to differences in type of surgery, surgical and anesthetic technique, physical examinations, and reporting. Perioperative hypotension can cause stroke by causing hypoperfusion of cerebral vascular *watershed* areas. Hypotension also can cause cerebral hypoperfusion in the setting of significant carotid stenosis.

Many investigators have reported that the most common type of stroke occurs within 2 to 5 days postoperatively. Common mechanisms include postoperative atrial fibrillation with thromboembolism, postoperative hypotension, carotid artery stenosis or plaque rupture, embolism related to surgical procedure (carotid or cardiac), and fat embolism.

It has been controversial as to whether or not the presence of carotid bruits preoperatively increases the risk of perioperative stroke. Studies have shown that the presence of an asymptomatic carotid bruit is associated with either no increased risk or only minimally increased risk of a perioperative stroke. The Asymptomatic Carotid Atherosclerosis Study (ACAS) showed no statistically significant difference in reduction of major strokes in patients who received prophylactic carotid endarterectomy before cardiac and vascular surgery. Prophylactic endarterectomy in this group of patients is not believed to be warranted at this time. Patients with a previous transient ischemic attack or stroke may be at higher risk for a perioperative stroke, but study results have been inconclusive.

A study by Wong et al[3] has shown that surgery and anesthesia are risks for stoke. The perioperative stroke rate was highest with cardiac, neurologic, and vascular procedures. It is hypothesized that changes in the coagulation system induced by surgery are responsible for a temporary hypercoagulable state, which predisposes to stroke. Postoperative changes, such as activation of coagulation and fibrinolysis, decreases in platelets, increases in factor VII activity and fibrinogen, and decreases in plasminogen, all have been observed and likely contribute to increased coagulability.

The present patient had a right middle cerebral artery stroke. He had a significant delay in postoperative physical therapy for his hip fracture because of his stroke. He had a subsequent decreased range of motion of the hip, likely related to the delay in therapy. The patient was transferred to a rehabilitation facility for completion of therapy. He eventually was able to use a wheeled walker after regaining partial strength in the left arm and leg.

Clinical Pearls

1. Hemorrhagic strokes are less common perioperatively than ischemic strokes and can be caused by a variety of factors, such as perioperative anticoagulation, severe hypertension, septic embolus, aneurysmal bleeding, hemorrhagic conversion of a bland infarct, and post–carotid endarterectomy hyperperfusion.

2. New-onset atrial fibrillation in the perioperative period is associated with an increased risk of stroke.

3. In the presence of a recent stroke or transient ischemic attack, surgery should be delayed for at least 6 to 12 weeks if possible.

REFERENCES:
1. Executive Committee for the Asymptomatic Carotid Atherosclerosis Trial: Endarterectomy for asymptomatic carotid artery stenosis. JAMA 273:1421–1428, 1995.
2. Limburg M, Wijdicks EFM, Li H: Ischemic stroke after surgical procedures. Neurology 50:895–901, 1998.
3. Wong GY, Warner DO, Schroeder DR, et al: Risk of surgery and anesthesia for ischemic stroke. Anesthesiology 92:425–432, 2000.
4. Kelley RE: Stroke in the postoperative period. Med Clin North Am. 85:1263–1276, 2001.

PATIENT 58

A 31-year-old man with intraoperative hemodynamic instability and fever

A 31-year-old man undergoes emergency surgery for a liver laceration sustained in a motorcycle accident. He has no known medical problems. In surgery, he develops tachycardia, hypotension, diaphoresis, muscular rigidity, and a fever.

Physical Examination: Temperature 105.2°F, pulse 120, respirations 14 (ventilated), blood pressure 88/52. Lungs: clear. Heart: tachycardia. No murmur. Musculoskeletal: significant diffuse rigidity, including trismus. Muscle fasciculations noted. Skin: diaphoretic, mottled.

Laboratory Findings: WBC 6,300/μL, hematocrit 27%, platelets 128,000/μL, Sodium 133 mEq/L, potassium 5.7 mEq/L, chloride 101 mEq/L, bicarbonate 20 mEq/L, BUN 31 mg/dL, creatinine 2.8 mg/dL, lactate 5.2 mEq/L, magnesium 3.5 mg/dL, creatine phosphokinase (CPK) 14,267 mg/dL, calcium 11.0 mg/dL.

Question: What caused the patient's instability?

Diagnosis: Malignant hyperthermia.

Discussion: Malignant hyperthermia is a potentially fatal disorder characterized by an exaggerated response to all inhalation anesthetics (except nitrous oxide) and the muscle relaxant succinylcholine. Implicated anesthetics include halothane, ethyl ether, cyclopropane, and methoxyflurane. The disorder has an autosomal dominant form and an autosomal recessive form; it also is associated with several types of myopathies.

Exposure to the offending agent causes release of calcium from muscle cell sarcoplasmic reticulum. The increased myoplasmic calcium triggers the metabolism of adenosine triphosphate to adenosine diphosphate phosphate, and heat. Other metabolic reactions include increased glycolysis and uncoupling of oxidative phosphorylation. Muscle contraction occurs; the accompanying fever is from the metabolic occurrences plus the muscle contraction. Also seen are increased oxygen consumption, carbon dioxide production, and muscle membrane disruption. These changes cause muscle rigidity, rhabdomyolysis, myoglobinuria, hyperkalemia , high fever, tachycardia, and hypotension. Fasciculations often are seen after administration of succinylcholine. The temperature can rise quickly (1°C every 5 minutes), sometimes reaching 107°F, but in some cases this has been a late finding. The presenting signs are tachypnea, tachycardia, and increased blood pressure from sympathetic nervous system stimulation secondary to hypermetabolism and hypercarbia. Muscle rigidity and fever quickly follow. Mottling of the skin with cyanosis and diaphoresis can be present. Other late findings include severe muscle swelling, pulmonary edema, disseminated intravascular coagulation, and acute renal failure.

Although some patients with the inherited susceptibility for malignant hyperthermia may have a chronic elevation of CPK or spontaneous muscle cramping, most are asymptomatic. It is important to question all patients about family history of intraoperative death, untoward responses to anesthesia, or a family history of any myopathy (e.g., muscular dystrophy or myotonia congenita).

The mainstay of treatment for malignant hyperthermia is dantrolene, which is a direct-acting skeletal muscle relaxant. It produces muscle relaxation by directly preventing the contractile response via inhibition of intracellular calcium release from myocyte endoplasmic reticulum.

As soon as malignant hyperthermia is recognized, the anesthetic should be stopped and surgery postponed. The patient should receive 100% oxygen (because of greatly increased oxygen requirements) and intravenous dantrolene, 1.0 to 2.5 mg/kg every 6 hours for at least 24 to 48 hours, until symptoms subside or until the patient can take oral dantrolene. Because ventricular tachycardia or ventricular fibrillation can occur, some physicians pretreat with procainamide. Calcium channel blockers should not be used during treatment for malignant hyperthermia; verapamil had been shown to interact with dantrolene to cause myocardial depression and hyperkalemia. CPK should be checked frequently, and urine should be observed for myoglobinuria. Appropriate therapy should be instituted for rhabdomyolysis, metabolic acidosis, and disseminated intravascular coagulation.

The present patient received immediate therapy with dantrolene and supportive measures. He had an initial response but developed recurrent symptoms requiring further infusions of dantrolene. His CPK rose to 24,231 mg/dL. He developed acute renal failure and required dialysis for fluid overload and hyperkalemia (potassium 6.5 mEq/L). The patient eventually improved and left the intensive care unit after 6 days.

Clinical Pearls

1. The incidence of malignant hyperthermia is 1:50,000 to 1:100,000.
2. To evaluate a patient for malignant hyperthermia, the gold standard is to test the response of a segment of biopsied muscle (from the vastus lateralis or vastus medialis) to caffeine or halothane and observe for contraction.
3. Drugs believed to be safe to use in patients susceptible to malignant hyperthermia include benzodiazepines, local anesthetics, opioids, ketamine, propofol, pancuronium, vecuronium, nitrous oxide, atracurium, and barbiturates.

REFERENCES

1. Dinarello CA, Gelfand JA: Fever and hyperthermia. In: Braunwald E, Fauci AS, Kasper DL et al (eds): Harrison's Principles of Internal Medicine, 15th ed. New York, McGraw-Hill, 2001, pp 90–94.
2. Rosenberg H, Fletcher JE, Brandom BW: Malignant hyperthermia and other pharmacogenetic disorders. In: Barash PG, Cullen BF, Stoelting RK (eds): Clinical Anesthesia, 4th ed. Philadelphia, Lippincott Williams & Wilkins, 2001, pp 521–530.
3. Physicians Desk Reference, 56th ed. Montvale, NJ, Medical Economics Company, 2002, pp 2887–2888.
4. Rosenberg H, Antognini JF, Muldoon, S: Testing for malignant hyperthermia. Anesthesiology 96:232–240, 2002.

PATIENT 59

A 64-year-old woman with postoperative shortness of breath

A 64-year-old woman with hypertension underwent a thyroidectomy and mediastinal dissection for papillary carcinoma of the thyroid. Her past medical history was notable for poorly controlled hypertension. Her only medication is enalapril. One day postoperatively, she develops shortness of breath, tachypnea, tachycardia, and hypoxia. Her oxygen saturation on 2 L of oxygen drops to 87%, and she has bilateral rales.

Physical Examination: Temperature 98.8°F, pulse 108, respirations 22, blood pressure 182/104. HEENT: normal. Neck: 3 cm jugular venous distention at 30°. Lungs: bilateral rales of the lower half of both lung fields. Heart: tachycardic. Normal S_1 and S_2, positive S_4. Abdomen: benign. Extremities: trace pretibial edema.

Laboratory Findings: WBC 8,600/μL, hematocrit 36.6%, platelets 205,000/μL. Sodium 137 mEq/L, potassium 3.9 mEq/L, chloride 100 mEq/L, bicarbonate 26 mEq/L, BUN 18 mg/dL, creatinine 1.6 mg/dL. Chest radiograph: moderate cardiomegaly and pulmonary congestion with cephalization and peribronchial cuffing. ECG: sinus rhythm with tachycardia. No ischemic changes. Prominent voltage in the precordial leads.

Question: What is the cause of the patient's postoperative hypoxia?

Diagnosis: Postoperative congestive heart failure (CHF) caused by diastolic dysfunction.

Discussion: Postoperative CHF has several possible causative factors. The most common cause is related to preexisting left ventricular dysfunction: perioperative changes in intravascular volumes, changes in afterload, the occurrence of perioperative ischemia, and catecholamine surges all can affect the already compromised ventricle, resulting in CHF. Causes of CHF in the presence of a normal left ventricle include perioperative ischemia, injudicious use of intravenous fluids, and lengthy surgical procedures. Studies also have shown that a history of dysrhythmias and diabetes predisposes to perioperative CHF. Diastolic dysfunction, characterized by normal left ventricular systolic function but decreased ventricular relaxation during diastole, also can predispose to perioperative CHF. The major cause of diastolic dysfunction is hypertension; on echocardiogram, hypertension-induced left ventricular hypertrophy often is seen. Positive inotropes (e.g., digoxin) should not be used in this condition because they can worsen symptoms. Medications such as calcium channel blockers, β-blockers, and angiotensin-converting enzyme inhibitors all have been helpful in treatment. Diuretics are useful when symptoms of pulmonary congestion are present. Perioperative worsening of diastolic dysfunction can be precipitated by worsening of hypertension and by increased intravascular volume.

For patients with preexisting CHF, cardiac function should be optimized preoperatively. If the evaluation of the CHF in the past did not include an echocardiogram, one should be obtained if possible to make the distinction between systolic and diastolic dysfunction. This distinction allows appropriate medication choices for subsequent treatment. Depending on the clinical situation, consideration also should be given to evaluating for silent coronary artery disease.

Studies have tried to determine if intraoperative hemodynamic monitoring is useful for patients with a history of CHF or ischemia. A randomized study by Bender et al[3] showed no difference in morbidity and mortality in patients undergoing vascular surgery who were given pulmonary artery catheters perioperatively. An American College of Physicians/American College of Cardiology/American Heart Association Task Force determined a few clinical conditions that may warrant the perioperative use of a pulmonary artery catheter, including recent myocardial infarction, unstable angina, symptomatic valvular disease, and refractory CHF, and certain types of high-risk situations, such as aortic surgeries, extensive intra-abdominal surgery, prostatic resection, and high-risk obstetric patients with cardiac disease.

For patients who take digoxin, the physician should be aware that the risk of digoxin toxicity can increase in the perioperative period. Multiple clinical factors can increase the risk of digoxin toxicity, including hypokalemia, hypomagnesemia, hypercalcemia, several anesthetic agents, and amiodarone. Studies have shown that withholding digoxin preoperatively can worsen CHF by a decrease in left ventricular ejection fraction, although a study by Mangano also has shown that digoxin increases the risk of perioperative ventricular tachycardia. For patients with mild, well-compensated CHF who are in sinus rhythm, the physician should consider holding the medication preoperatively and titrating diuretics and angiotensin-converting enzyme inhibitors. For patients who require digoxin perioperatively, the serum level should be checked to ensure it is in the appropriate therapeutic range.

The present patient had never had an episode of CHF before this surgery. Evaluation of her fluid balance found her to be 2 L positive. Cardiac enzymes and an ECG revealed no ischemia. An echocardiogram revealed moderate left ventricular concentric hypertrophy, suggestive of diastolic dysfunction. The patient was treated with two doses of a diuretic and the addition of a calcium channel blocker to her medication regimen. She did well and was discharged home.

Clinical Pearls

1. It has not been determined what role transesophageal echocardiography should play intraoperatively in patients with left ventricular dysfunction.
2. Digoxin-induced dysrhythmias can be treated with phenytoin or lidocaine. The addition of magnesium also has been found to be helpful. Life-threatening digoxin toxicity should be treated with digoxin Fab antibody fragments.
3. Patients with postoperative CHF should be evaluated for ischemia, new dysrhythmia, and volume overload.

REFERENCES

1. Mangano DT: Perioperative cardiac morbidity. Anesthesiology 72:153–184, 1990.
2. Guidelines for perioperative cardiovascular evaluation for noncardiac surgery: Report of the American College of Cardiology/American Heart Association Task Force on Practice Guidelines (Committee on Perioperative Cardiovascular Evaluation of Noncardiac Surgery). J Am Coll Cardiol 27:910–948, 1996.
3. Bender JS, Smith-Meek MA, Jones CE: Routine pulmonary artery catheterization does not reduce morbidity and mortality of elective vascular surgery: Results of a prospective, randomized trial. Ann Surg 229–237, 1997.
4. Falcone RA, Ziegelstein RC: Cardiovascular disease and hypertension. In: Gross RJ, Caputo GM (eds): Kammerer and Gross Medical Consultation, 3rd ed. Baltimore, Williams & Williams, 1998, pp 149–206.
5. Harrision GG, Opie LH: Heart failure and its therapy in the perioperative period. In: Foex P, Harrison GG, Opie LH (eds): Cardiovascular Drugs in the Perioperative Period. Philadelphia, Lippincott-Raven Publishers, 1999, pp 278–305.

PATIENT 60

A 40-year-old man with fever and confusion

A 40-year-old man is brought to the hospital with a 2-day history of incontinence, confusion, and stiffness. His medical history is notable for paranoid schizophrenia and hypertension. His medications are thioridazine and nifedipine. In the emergency department, he is found to be obtunded, with significant rigidity of his limbs and unstable vital signs.

Physical Examination: Temperature 105°F, pulse 110, respirations 24, blood pressure 162/106. General appearance: Diaphoretic, stuporous, responsive to pain. Heart and lungs normal. Neurologic: obtunded, responsive to pain. Trismus present. Extremities rigid; deep tendon reflexes difficult to elicit.

Laboratory Findings: WBC 14,400/μL, hematocrit 41%, platelets 338,000/μL. Electrolytes normal. Lactate dehydrogenase 738 mg/dL, creatine phosphokinase 10,315 mg/dL, alkaline phosphate 300, alanine aminotransferase 96 mg/dL, aspartate aminotransferase 85 mg/dL.

Question: What is the cause of the patient's symptom complex?

Diagnosis: Neuroleptic malignant syndrome (NMS) in a patient on antipsychotic medication.

Discussion: NMS is the most serious hazard of using **neuroleptic medication;** it occurs in approximately 1.5% of all patients taking these drugs and has a 20% mortality rate. Because of the high mortality rate and because it can be confused with other clinical entities, clinicians should be familiar with its typical presentations.

NMS is an idiosyncratic reaction to neuroleptics that can occur at any time after initiation of such medications. It develops more commonly in men, patients with organic brain syndromes, and patients receiving neuroleptics by depot injection. The high-potency neuroleptics are associated more frequently with the development of NMS, but all neurologic medications carry the risk.

The syndrome is thought to be caused by changes in thermoregulation induced by neuroleptic dopamine receptor blockade in the basal ganglia and hypothalamus. The result is increased heat generation via muscle contraction and reduced heat dissipation. The neurologic and autonomic changes in NMS are thought to be due to abnormalities in neurotransmission in dopaminergic striatal and hypothalamic neurons. The signs and symptoms of NMS are listed in the top table. The clinical syndrome often evolves over a few days. Autonomic signs and symptoms are common, especially tachypnea, tachycardia, and labile blood pressure. The level of consciousness is variable; some patients may remain alert, but the most severely afflicted develop stupor and coma.

The differential diagnosis is broad (see bottom table). In particular, heatstroke and catatonia can mimic NMS. Heatstroke is characterized by hyperpyrexia, tachycardia, and a decreased level of consciousness. It can be distinguished from NMS by dry skin, in contrast to the diaphoresis that can be seen in NMS, and flaccid rather than rigid muscles. Catatonia shares with NMS the clinical features of mutism and muscular rigidity. The waxy flexibility and cataplexy of catatonia are not features of NMS.

The mainstay of treatment includes immediate discontinuation of all psychotropic medications; antipyretic therapy; stabilization of blood pressure; and treatment of secondary abnormalities, such as rhabdomyolysis, renal insufficiency, and fluid and electrolyte imbalances. Antipyretic therapy includes acetaminophen plus cooling blankets. Dantrolene also should be given; it is a direct-acting skeletal muscle relaxant that works by inhibiting intracellular calcium release from myocyte endoplasmic reticulum, thereby decreasing muscle contraction and decreasing thermogenesis. Amantadine or bromocriptine also can be tried if the patient does not respond to other measures. Both agents help reverse the central dopamine receptor blockade caused by neuroleptic medications. With institution of the aforementioned measures, resolution of symptoms still can take 10 days or longer.

The present patient had a poor response to therapy consisting of intravenous fluids, oxygen, acetaminophen, cooling blanket, and dantrolene. He required ventilatory support and intermittent antihypertensive medication. His temperature remained at 104° to 106°F, he developed rhabdomyolysis and acute renal failure, and he died as a result of cardiac arrest after development of ventricular tachycardia.

Common Clinical Features of Neuroleptic
Malignant Syndrome

Hyperthermia (temperatures 102–107°F)
Rigidity
Dyskinesias
Akinesia
Trismus
Dystonia
Tremor
Opisthotonos
Seizures
Positive Babinski signs
Altered consciousness (mutism, stupor, obtundation, coma)
Autonomic abnormalities (sialorrhea, diaphoresis, incontinence, tachypnea, tachycardia, labile blood pressure)

Differential Diagnosis

Catatonia
Infection
Heatstroke
Malignant hyperthermia
Seizures
Toxins (tetanus, strychnine, curare, botulism, phencyclidine)
Hypocalcemic tetany
Pellagra

Clinical Pearls

1. The symptom complex of NMS closely resembles that of malignant hyperthermia; they likely have a similar pathophysiology.

2. Patients with a history of NMS may be at higher risk for developing malignant hyperthermia when undergoing surgical procedures.

3. Long-term use of neuroleptic medications is associated with tardive dyskinesia, characterized by involuntary choreoathetoid movements that often involve orofacial muscles. The syndrome is thought to be due to supersensitivity of dopamine receptors that have been chronically blocked.

REFERENCES

1. Lazarus A: Neuroleptic malignant syndrome: Detection and management. Psych Ann 15:706–712, 1985.
2. Holleran DK, Ziring BS: Medical evaluation of the patient with psychiatric illness. In: Merli GJ, Weitz HH (eds): Medical Management of the Surgical Patient, 2nd ed. Philadelphia, WB Saunders Company, 1998, pp 351–358.

PATIENT 61

An 81-year-old woman with ascending cholangitis and choledocholithiasis

An 81-year-old woman is admitted with fever and right upper quadrant pain. She is found to have ascending cholangitis, significant cholelithiasis, and choledocholithiasis. She undergoes an endoscopic retrograde cholangiopancreatography with sphincterotomy, but the common bile duct stone is not able to be extracted. She receives percutaneous stenting of the bile duct and is scheduled for an open cholecystectomy with common bile duct exploration.

Physical Examination: Temperature 100.5°F, pulse 96, respirations 18, blood pressure 136/80. HEENT: unremarkable. Chest: clear. Heart: regular rhythm. Grade II/VI systolic ejection murmur at the left sternal border, grade II/VI holosystolic murmur at the apex radiating to the axilla. Abdomen: soft, hypoactive bowel sounds, no masses, tender to palpation in the right upper quadrant and epigastrium with involuntary guarding but no rebound.

Laboratory Findings: WBC 17,400/μL, hematocrit 36.9%, platelets 215,000/μL. Sodium 146 mEq/L, potassium 3.3 mEq/L, chloride 107 mEq/L, bicarbonate 22 mEq/L, BUN 32 mg/dL, creatinine 1.4 mg/dL. Total bilirubin 2.4 mg/dL, alkaline phosphatase 408 mg/dL, aspartate aminotransferase 121 mg/dL, alanine aminotransferase 168 mg/dL. Amylase and lipase normal.

Question: What are the major concerns in preparing a geriatric patient for surgery?

Answer: Geriatric patients are at increased risk for cardiac and pulmonary complications in the perioperative period, and are also at greater risk for delirium.

Discussion: There are currently >33 million people in the United States who are >65 years old. It has been estimated that by 2030 this number will increase to 35 million people; one fourth of those will be >85 years old. Individuals >65 years old have the highest rate of surgery and the highest rate of surgical complications. Dealing effectively with perioperative issues in the elderly is crucial to ensuring a functional lifestyle for this segment of the population.

Studies have evaluated predictors of postoperative morbidity and mortality in the elderly. Liu and Leung studied the outcomes of 410 surgical procedures and found the following to be predictors of postoperative morbidity: history of arrhythmias, congestive heart failure, neurologic disease, urgent or emergent surgery, and intraoperative vasopressor use. They did not find age, American Society of Anesthesiologists classification, number of comorbid conditions, or type of surgery to be predictive of adverse postoperative events. Predictors of postoperative death were a history of coronary artery disease, congestive heart failure, neurologic disease, and intraoperative vasopressor use. Polanczyk et al found that advanced age was associated with a higher risk of perioperative cardiogenic pulmonary edema, myocardial infarction, ventricular arrhythmias, pneumonia, respiratory failure, and death. The combined rates of all types of major perioperative complications according to age are shown in the table. Perioperative mortality rates were greater in patients ≥80 years old (2.6%) compared with patients <80 years old (0.7%).

Perioperative Complications Based on Age

Age Range (y)	Complication Rates (%)
≤59	4.3
60–69	5.7
70–79	9.6
≥80	12.5

Adapted from Polanczyk CA, Marcantonio E, Goldman L, et al: Impact of age on perioperative complications and length of stay in patients undergoing noncardiac surgery. Ann Intern Med 134:637–643, 2001.

In performing perioperative assessment of the elderly, the clinician should be mindful of the problems unique to this group, including higher prevalence of cardiovascular disease, malnutrition, and poor functional status and age-related changes in renal and hepatic function, an increased risk of medication side effects, and an increased risk of delirium. The risk of death increases significantly in the 60s and 70s and is related mainly to the high age-related prevalence of cardiovascular disease. Some studies have linked poor functional capacity in the elderly with a higher risk of perioperative cardiac events. The mechanism is not clear. It is prudent to consider noninvasive cardiac testing preoperatively for elderly patients who cannot perform at least 4 METs of work, especially if they are to undergo moderate-to-high stress surgery and if they have multiple cardiac risk factors. In addition, elderly patients have a higher propensity for silent cardiac events, especially in the presence of diabetes. Postoperative ischemia or infarction in the elderly may present in an atypical fashion, for example, as confusion or decreased urine output, without any chest pain or chest pressure.

The nutritional status of elderly patients often is compromised. Albumin should be measured because protein malnutrition often effects wound healing. Calcium, magnesium, phosphate, and potassium should be evaluated and repleted as necessary. If there is an anemia out of proportion to the underlying illness, iron stores should be evaluated.

Elderly patients have age-related decrements in pulmonary, cardiac, hepatic, and renal function. One study showed that postoperative pulmonary complications were more common than postoperative cardiac complications. Renal function declines with age; studies have shown a decrease in glomerular filtration rate of 6% to 8% per decade. This problem is compounded if patients have superimposed hypertension, diabetes, or vascular disease. Anesthetic agents and other perioperative medications take a longer time for elimination. There also is a mild age-related decrease in hepatic function, which results in decreased rates of drug clearance. An additional problem is polypharmacy in the elderly. The use of multiple medications can produce additive or antagonistic actions and can complicate anesthetic management and cause unpredictability in drug pharmacokinetics.

Postoperative delirium in the elderly is a common problem. The biggest risk factor is preexisting dementia, possibly because this may increase neurologic vulnerability to ischemic injury from perioperative hypoperfusion. Other risk factors, such as infection, medication side effects, and metabolic abnormalities, have been identified. Current trials are evaluating whether or not the use of donepezil (Aricept) perioperatively helps reduce the incidence of postoperative confusion.

Elderly patients commonly have a muted physiologic response to illness, particularly infection. Patients may not mount a fever or a leukocytosis in response to infection and may not mount a tachycardia even in the face of shock. Physicians should have a low threshold to evaluate for postoperative infection.

A high index of suspicion should be maintained for perioperative complications in elderly patients. A wide range of abnormalities, such as hypoxia, ischemia, infection, and metabolic abnormalities, may present in a subdued fashion, sometimes only as a change in mental status.

The present patient underwent subsequent open cholecystectomy with common bile duct exploration. She tolerated the surgery but was delirious postoperatively. Her course was complicated by a right lower lobe pneumonia, which was treated by antibiotics. Her delirium took several days to improve; by postoperative day 10, she was transferred to an acute rehabilitation facility and was still experiencing sundowning in the evening. She also had significant hypoalbuminemia with peripheral edema and partial dehiscence of her surgical wound. It took 10 weeks for the patient to recover.

Clinical Pearls

1. Although perioperative morbidity and mortality in elderly patients are greater than in younger patients, they are not prohibitively high if coexisting medical problems are stable.

2. Some studies have shown a decreased risk of postoperative delirium in elderly patients receiving regional rather than general anesthesia.

3. Studies of elderly patients undergoing cardiac surgery show a mortality rate of 1.9% to 20%, depending on age and type of procedure. Patients ≥ 81 years old undergoing mitral valve repair or combined aortic and mitral valve replacement had the highest death rate at 20%.

REFERENCES

1. Gerson MC, Hurst JM, Hertzberg VS, et al: Cardiac prognosis in noncardiac geriatric surgery. Ann Intern Med 103:832–837, 1985.
2. Aziz S, Grover FL: Cardiovascular surgery in the elderly. Cardiol Clin 17:213–232, 1999.
3. Liu LL, Leung JM: Predicting adverse postoperative outcomes in patients aged 80 years and older. J Am Geriatri Soc 48:405–412, 2000.
4. Muravchick S: Preoperative assessment of the elderly patient. Anesth Clin North Am 18:71–89, 2000.
5. Polanczyk CA, Marcantonio E, Goldman L, et al: Impact of age on perioperative complications and length of stay in patients undergoing noncardiac surgery. Ann Intern Med 134:637–643, 2001.

PATIENT 62

A 27-year-old woman with a seizure disorder requiring general anesthesia

A 27-year-old woman with history of tonic-clonic seizures requires general anesthesia for a tubal ligation. She has seizures approximately once every 2 months despite the use of carbamazepine, phenytoin, and topiramate. In the recovery room, she has a prolonged tonic-clonic seizure.

Physical Examination: Vital signs: normal. General appearance: somnolent but arousable and oriented. HEENT: gingival hyperplasia. Lungs: clear. Heart: normal. Abdomen: sutures at surgical site intact.

Laboratory Findings: CBC: normal. Electrolytes: normal. Phenytoin level 16.2 mg/dL (therapeutic range 10 to 20 mg/dL). Carbamazepine level 3.2 mg/dL (therapeutic range 6 to 10 mg/dL).

Question: What are the risks of a perioperative seizure in patients with seizure disorders?

Answer: For patients with poorly controlled epilepsy, there is a small risk of seizure during stages I and II (excitation and delirium) of anesthesia. The risk of seizure after neurosurgery depends on the type of procedure, and can range from 25% to as high as 80%.

Discussion: Patients with known seizure disorders should have their seizures as well controlled as possible before surgery. They should have medication levels checked to ensure that the levels are in the therapeutic range. Patients should take their usual medication the morning of the procedure, then restart the medication postoperatively as soon as possible because decreasing levels of antiseizure medication can increase the risk of postoperative seizures.

Clinical entities other than a primary seizure disorder should be considered in certain circumstances. Severe postoperative hyponatremia can cause seizures. Young women have been noted to be especially susceptible to postoperative syndrome of inappropriate antidiuretic hormone with severe hyponatremia. Any woman with postoperative seizures should have an immediate serum sodium level checked. Alcohol or drug withdrawal can present as postoperative seizures. Alcohol-related seizures usually occur 8 to 48 hours after the last alcoholic intake.

Most anesthetic medications have been implicated in causing seizure activity, although for the most part, such occurrences are rare. Ketamine has been shown to cause seizure activity occasionally, and although it has been used safely in most seizure patients, it is prudent to use another agent. Enflurane has been shown to increase spike and wave activity on electroencephalograms in children, especially in the setting of hypocarbia. Enflurane likely should be avoided in seizure patients.

Some anticonvulsants have interaction with anesthetic medications. Most notably, phenytoin and carbamazepine can cause resistance to the action of nondepolarizing neuromuscular blocking agents. Phenobarbital can induce hepatic microsomal enzymes; this causes increased metabolism and dose requirements of a variety of anesthetic drugs, such as the halogenated volatile agents.

The present patient had a history of inadequately controlled seizures; the fact that her carbamazepine level was subtherapeutic likely contributed to her seizure. Her seizure was treated successfully with diazepam. She received a partial loading dose of carbamazepine as soon as she could take oral medication. She developed a moderate bilateral aspiration pneumonitis, consistent with aspiration during her seizure. She was given supportive treatment and made a full recovery.

Clinical Pearls

1. Postoperative seizures can damage the fresh surgical wound as a result of the force of seizure-related muscle contractions.

2. Patients experiencing postoperative seizures should be monitored for the development of aspiration pneumonitis and pneumonia.

3. Many types of neurosurgery have postoperative seizure as a potential complication; such patients are treated with prophylactic anticonvulsants.

REFERENCES

1. Arieff AI: Hyponatremia, convulsions, respiratory arrest, and permanent brain damage after elective surgery in healthy women. N Engl J Med 314:1529–1535, 1986.
2. Arar MG, Dairi Y, Corman LC: Perioperative management of neurologic conditions and complications. In: Gross RJ, Caputo GM (eds): Kammerer and Gross Medical Consultation, 3rd ed. Baltimore, Williams & Wilkins, 1998, pp 553–556.
3. Dierdorf SF: Anesthesia for patients with rare and coexisting diseases. In: Barash PG, Cullen BF, Stoelting RK (eds): Clinical Anesthesia, 4th ed. Philadelphia, Lippincott Williams & Wilkins, 2001, pp 491–520.

PATIENT 63

A 75-year-old man with confusion and lethargy after a transurethral resection of the prostate

A 75-year-old man underwent a transurethral resection of the prostate (TURP) for prostatic enlargement after recurrence of prostate cancer. The cancer had been treated several years prior with radiation therapy. He is otherwise healthy; his medications are tamsulosin (Flomax) and atorvastatin (Lipitor). Intraoperatively, he developed hypertension (188/105 mmHg) with bradycardia. Immediately postoperatively, he develops hypotension, confusion, lethargy, nausea, and vomiting.

Physical Examination: General appearance: obtunded, oriented to person only, complaining of nausea and blurred vision. Temperature 99.2°F, pulse 88, respirations 18, blood pressure 90/56. HEENT: pupils sluggish. Fundi: normal. Neck: 2-cm jugular venous distention. Lungs: rales bilaterally 3 up from lung bases. Heart: regular rate and rhythm with some ectopic beats, positive S_3. Abdomen: benign. Neurologic: obtunded. Moves all four limbs to pain. Reflexes 2+ throughout. Toes downgoing.

Laboratory Findings: Serum sodium 113 mEq/L, potassium 3.3 mEq/L, serum osmolality 256 mmol/L.

Question: What is the main cause of confusion after TURP?

Answer: Profound hyponatremia and glycine toxicity.

Discussion: Benign prostatic hypertrophy affects 12% of men > 65 years old. Of all men who live to age 80, an estimated 20% to 30% undergo prostatectomy. Currently, 400,000 TURPs are done in United States each year. This number is expected to increase progressively over the next several years as the population ages.

In general, TURP is considered to be a fairly safe procedure in that the mortality is low (0.2% to 0.8%). Perioperative morbidity ranges from 7% to 20%, however. The major risks are listed in the table below. The procedure itself involves insertion of a resectoscope through the urethra and resection of prostatic tissue with a cutting-coagulating metal loop. Large amounts of irrigating solution are required during the procedure, and the solution is moderately hypotonic to maintain its transparency. In the past, water was used, which caused acute severe hypo-osmolality with massive hemolysis. Currently the most commonly used irrigating solutions are glycine, mannitol, sorbitol, and glucose.

Complications of Transurethral Resection of the Prostate

Bladder perforation or rupture
Hypovolemia
Cardiac ischemia or infarct
Sepsis
Coagulopathy
Hemolysis
Pulmonary edema
Deep venous thrombosis
TURP syndrome

The most common morbid event is the development of the TURP syndrome; this refers to complications that arise from absorption of irrigation fluid into the intravascular space. It occurs in 2% to 15% of patients. It can present in a variety of ways; the major associated signs and symptoms are shown below. During surgery, the irrigation solution can be absorbed intravascularly via the prostatic plexus and can be absorbed more slowly via the retroperitoneal and perivesical spaces. The amount of irrigating solution absorbed depends on the height of the container of solution above the patient (which determines the hydrostatic pressure) and the duration of surgery.

TURP syndrome has a variety of components and is the hemodynamic and neurologic consequence of the absorption of large amounts of hypotonic irrigation fluid. It has been reported as soon as 15 minutes after the start of the resection and as late as 24 hours postoperatively. Rapid absorption of irrigant (rates of 200 mL/min have been noted) can cause sudden hypertension with a reflex bradycardia. Subsequent intravascular fluid shifts can cause postoperative intravascular hypovolemia and hypotension.

Severe hyponatremia seen in TURP syndrome can cause nausea, vomiting, headache, confusion, encephalopathy, pulmonary edema, cardiovascular collapse, seizure, and death. Decreases in serum sodium < 125 mmol/L have been reported in 15% of cases and can occur rapidly (within 15 minutes of initiation of irrigant use).

The hypo-osmolality caused by absorption of irrigant is thought to cause cerebral edema, with resultant neurologic abnormalities. It is not the hyponatremia that causes the cerebral dysfunction, but rather the hypo-osmolality with movement of the free water across the blood-brain barrier. It also can cause reflex hypertension and bradycardia (the *Cushing reflex*).

Treatment of hyponatremia is controversial. For mild hyponatremia, fluid restriction is adequate; for severe symptomatic hyponatremia, a loop diuretic with or without concurrent 3% saline may be necessary. Some authors believe that loop diuretics can worsen hyponatremia by causing salt wasting, but generally water is lost in excess of sodium; any lost sodium can be given back to the patient with administration of 3% saline.

A complication of glycine absorption is increase of serum ammonia with resultant changes in cerebral function. Signs and symptoms of glycine toxicity include nausea, vomiting, headache, malaise,

Signs and Symptoms of TURP Syndrome

Nausea/vomiting	Blindness	Hypotension
Headache	Coma	Hypertension
Confusion	Hyponatremia	Bradycardia
Seizures	Hypo-osmolality	Dysrhythmia
Lethargy	High ammonia levels	Pulmonary edema
Paralysis	Hemolysis	Cardiovascular shock
Dilated unreactive pupils	Acute renal failure	Death

and weakness. The various visual changes associated with TURP syndrome (ranging from blurred vision to transient blindness) are thought to be secondary to glycine toxicity.

The present patient suffered from the neurologic and cardiovascular effects of TURP syndrome. He was given furosemide (Lasix) to help correct the hyponatremia and to treat the congestive heart failure. He received 3% saline in small amounts over several hours (in amounts equal to what he had lost in urine over the preceding hours). His serum sodium was raised to 128 mEq/L over 16 hours, then to 135 mEq/L over the subsequent 24 hours. The congestive heart failure resolved, and his mental status normalized. In acute hyponatremia, experts recommend that serum sodium be corrected at a rate of 1 to 2 mmol/L per hour. For chronic hyponatremia, it should be corrected at only 0.5 to 1.0 mmol/L per hour. To avoid central pontine myelinolysis, experts recommend a maximal increase in serum sodium of only 12 mmol/L per day, even in acute hyponatremia.

Clinical Pearls

1. When serum sodium decreases rapidly to <120 mEq/L, it has a negative inotropic effect on the heart, with possible subsequent hypotension and congestive heart failure. The ECG can develop widened QRS complexes and ventricular ectopy.

2. The use of regional anesthesia for TURP provides the advantage of allowing evaluation of the patient's mental status, which may reflect early TURP syndrome.

3. Regional anesthesia for TURP also results in sympathetic blockade, which can increase venous capacitance and decrease the effect of excess fluid absorption.

REFERENCES
1. Mebust WK, Holtgrewe HL, Cockett ATK, et al: Transurethral prostatectomy: Immediate and postoperative complications: A cooperative study of 13 participating institutions evaluating 3885 patients. J Urol 141:243–247, 1989.
2. Gravenstein D: Transurethral resection of the prostate (TURP) syndrome: A review of pathophysiology and management. Anesth Analg 84:438–446, 1997.
3. Medina JJ, Parra RO, Moore RG: Benign prostatic hyperplasia (the aging prostate). Med Clin North Am 83:1213–1229, 1999.
4. Malhotra V: Transurethral resection of the prostate. Anesth Clin North Am 18:883–897, 2000.

PATIENT 64

A 48-year-old woman with questions about general versus regional anesthesia

A 48-year-old woman is about to undergo resection of an ovarian mass that is suspicious for ovarian cancer. Years prior, she had had epidural anesthesia for childbirth that resulted in a *wet tap* (accidental dural puncture with loss of significant cerebrospinal fluid) requiring a blood patch. She is nervous about any subsequent attempts at regional anesthesia and wants to know the pros and cons of general versus regional anesthesia.

Question: What are the major risks of regional anesthesia?

Answer: The major risks are hypotension and bradycardia. Neurologic injuries are uncommon.

Discussion: Whether to use general versus regional (neuraxial) anesthesia depends on a variety of factors, including type of surgery; positioning required; duration of surgery; preference of surgeon, anesthesiologist, and patient; and existing medical conditions. The most common side effects of neuraxial anesthesia are hypotension and bradycardia related to the blockade of sympathetic efferents. This blockade can cause a potential decrease in coronary perfusion pressure but can be managed by performing a *controlled spinal* (a slow induction, which generally limits the degree of hypotension). Regional anesthesia can be useful for patients with severe pulmonary disease when intubation needs to be avoided. Some studies have found an increased incidence of confusion with general anesthesia compared with neuraxial techniques, but more recent studies have found no difference between the two. Many studies have shown that there are no differences in cardiac morbidity and mortality between patients receiving regional versus general anesthesia.

Neurologic injuries are uncommon during and after neuraxial anesthesia. A prospective survey showed that of 103,730 regional anesthetics, there were only 34 complications, and 19 of those resulted in complete recovery within 3 months.

The incidence of neurologic dysfunction from hemorrhagic complications associated with neuraxial anesthesia is estimated <1:150,000 epidural and 1:220,000 spinal anesthesias. In some of these patients, the needle or catheter insertions were difficult or bloody; other patients had evidence of a hemostatic abnormality. In still others, spinal hematoma had developed because of the use of heparin around the time of neuraxial anesthesia. Direct nerve injury also is rare and has been estimated to occur in <1:10,000 neuraxial anesthesias.

There is evidence that anesthetic agents themselves are neurotoxic. Patients have developed cauda equina syndrome after single-dose and continuous spinal anesthesia and intrathecal injection during extended epidural anesthesia and repeated intrathecal injection with lidocaine. One practitioner advocates avoidance of >60 mg of lido-

caine and avoidance of the use of epinephrine to prolong the action of the lidocaine.

A large study has shown neuraxial anesthesia to be safe in patients on antiplatelet agents. If a patient is receiving more than one antiplatelet agent, the risks are unknown. For patients on long-term warfarin, their the international normalized ratio should be in the normal range before neuraxial anesthesia is attempted.

The most common complication of neuraxial anesthesia is the postdural puncture headache (the *spinal headache*). This headache is beleived to be due to persistent leak through a dural hole or tear, resulting in a lowering of cerebrospinal fluid pressure in the spinal canal. This decreased pressure causes downward traction on the structures of the central nervous system with a resultant postural headache. Severe headaches that do not resolve after 5 to 10 days of bed rest and analgesics can be treated with an epidural blood patch; 50% of these headaches resolve within 5 days and 90% within 10 days. The use of a blood patch involves injection of 20 ml of the patient's own blood under sterile technique into the epidural space in the area of the epidural tear to prevent further cerebrospinal fluid leakage. Some practitioners also try 300 to 500 mg of intravenous caffeine, which is thought to increase cerebrospinal fluid production. The use of a blood patch is safe and has an efficacy of about 90% to 95%.

Other postoperative complications of neuraxial anesthesia include urinary retention, owing to blockade of the S2 and S4 sacral nerve roots; back pain from local tissue irritation or muscle spasm; and, rarely, epidural abscess. The incidence of epidural abscess is exceedingly low; depending on the study, the risk is between 0 and 3:65,000 anesthetics.

The present patient had received a blood patch after her dural puncture in the past. Because of this puncture, the anesthesiologist stated that the anesthetic coverage with another epidural may be *patchy*. The anesthesiologist thought that given her anxiety and the chance of an incomplete anesthetic, the patient should receive general anesthesia.

Clinical Pearls

1. The primary care provider should never recommend the method of anesthesia to the anesthesiologist.

2. Initial treatment of postdural puncture headaches should consist of analgesics, intravenous fluids, and bed rest. Intravenous caffeine or moderate oral caffeine intake also may be helpful because it may increase cerebrospinal fluid production.

3. When using low-molecular-weight heparin, the last dose of the medication should be given 12 hours before neuraxial anesthesia is performed. Subsequent dosing should not occur for at least 2 hours after the removal of the epidural catheter.

REFERENCES

1. Higgins TL: The changing profile of anesthetic practice: An update for internists. Cleve Clin J Med 60:219–232, 1993.
2. Bode RH, Lewis KP, Zarich SW, et al: Cardiac outcome after peripheral vascular surgery: Comparison of general and regional anesthesia. Anesthesiology 84:3–13, 1996
3. Neuraxial anesthesia and anticoagulation. American Society of Regional Anesthesia Consensus Conference, May 1998.
4. Spiekermann BF, Sibell DM, DiFazio C: Regional anesthesia In: Stone DJ, Bogdonoff DL, Leisure GS, et al (eds): Perioperative Care. St. Louis, Mosby, 1998, pp 693–770.
5. Horlocker TT: Complications of spinal and epidural anesthesia. Anesthesiol Clin North Am 18:407–428, 2000.

PATIENT 65

A 45-year-old man with a prosthetic valve who requires a partial lobectomy

A 45-year-old man with a prosthetic valve in the mitral positit-ion requires a partial lobectomy for lung cancer. He has a tilting-disk type of valve and his international normalized ratio (INR) is maintained between 2.5 and 3.5. For the purposes of the surgery, he will need his anticoagulation reversed.

Physical Examination: Vital signs: normal. Lungs: scant rales in the right midlung field. Heart: regular rate and rhythm. Mechanical S_1, normal S_2; no murmur, rub, or gallop.

Laboratory Findings: INR 2.9. Electrolytes normal. CBC normal.

Question: What are the thromboembolic risks of reversing anticoagulation perioperatively?

Answer: They vary widely with the clinical setting.

Discussion: Long-term **anticoagulation** is used to manage a wide variety of clinical conditions such as venous thromboembolism, hypercoagulable states, mechanical heart valves, cardiomyopathy, atrial fibrillation, dialysis grafts, and peripheral vascular disease. When such patients undergo surgery, they require appropriate perioperative management of their anticoagulation.

When long-term anticoagulation is not used, the risk of a thrombotic complication varies with the clinical setting. For example, the risk of thromboembolism in atrial fibrillation patients who are not anticoagulated is approximately 3% to 11% per year, with variation based on the patient's individual clinical characteristics, such as gender, hypertension, and coexistent valvular disease or cardiomyopathy. Patients with prosthetic heart valves have rates of thrombosis that depend on the type of prosthesis and the location (aortic versus mitral) of the valve. The first-generation caged ball valves and mitral position of the valve have been associated with the highest risk of thrombosis. The reported risk of thromboembolism per year in the absence of anticoagulation ranges from 8% to 22%.

For patients with prosthetic heart valves, it has long been observed that valves in the mitral position are more thrombotic than valves in the aortic position. First-generation caged-ball valves are more thrombogenic than the newer second-generation valves, such as the bileaflet and tilting disk valves. Bioprosthetic valves are the least thrombogenic. There is a paucity of data on rates of perioperative thromboembolic events, but Spandorfer[6] estimated a risk of 0.8% to 0.36% for 4 to 6 days of subtherapeutic INR.

It now is becoming common practice to stop warfarin 4 to 5 days preoperatively for patients with mechanical valves and to substitute low-molecular-weight heparin in the immediate perioperative period. The safety of this method has not yet been documented in the literature, so some practitioners still use conventional heparin, especially in patients with aortic and mitral prosthetic valves.

One of the most common clinical indications for long-term anticoagulation is atrial fibrillation. It has been stated in the ACC/AHA/ESC guidelines[4] that for patients without coexistent mechanical heart valves, anticoagulation can be stopped safely for 1 week without concomitant use of perioperative heparin. This statement is predicated on the fact that the average risk of thromboembolism in atrial fibrillation is 4% to 5% per year; given that, 1 week of no anticoagulation offers a miniscule risk. Jacobs and Nus-

baum[5] pointed out, however, that the surgical patient is in an inherently prothrombotic state and that changes in factors II, VII, IX, and X and proteins C and S induced by stopping and starting warfarin may predispose patients to a much greater thromboembolic risk. Some studies have shown a temporary hypercoagulable state, or *rebound phenomenon,* after stopping warfarin, but many others have seen no clinical prothrombotic effect.

The highest risk of thromboembolism perioperatively is seen in the following circumstances: recent deep venous thrombosis (within the past month), first-generation prosthetic heart valves, atrial fibrillation with a history of stroke or multiple risks for stroke, and a hypercoagulable state with recent thrombosis or history of life-threatening thrombosis. For patients receiving anticoagulation for venous thromboembolism, discontinuation of warfarin perioperatively is associated with a greater risk of thromboembolism than with discontinuation of warfarin for other reasons. Factors intrinsic to the surgical state, such as stasis from anesthesia and bed rest, and initiation of the coagulation cascade from disrupted tissue (with potential release of tissue thromboplastin and exposure of subendothelial collagen) likely play a role. Some patients may be affected by the rebound phenomenon mentioned previously. For patients with a recent thrombus, surgery should be delayed for at least 3 months to avoid recurrence.

When discontinuing warfarin preoperatively, an INR in the range of 2 to 3 takes 4 to 5 days to decrease to <1.5. Because of a slower rate of elimination, it may take longer in the elderly. The acceptable level of INR depends on the type of surgery and the type of anesthesia (regional versus general). Also, individual physicians differ as to their level of comfort. In any surgery associated with an increased risk of bleeding or in which bleeding would be disastrous (i.e., neurosurgery), the surgeon may insist on an INR of 1.0 or 1.1. Other surgeons are comfortable with an INR of ≤1.5. There are no data available that specifically measure the risk at each level. Likewise, the INR at which the anesthesiologist may feel comfortable using neuraxial anesthesia varies, but generally it is <1.3. For patients on warfarin requiring urgent surgery, subcutaneous vitamin K can reverse the INR in 8 to 10 hours. Oral vitamin K takes 18 to 24 hours to take effect; intravenous vitamin K can cause anaphylaxis and so should be avoided if possible. For an INR of 2 to 3, a subcutaneous dose of 1 to 2 mg of vitamin K is generally adequate. When surgery must be done emergently, 2 to 3 U of fresh frozen plasma can be used depending on the INR, followed by retesting of the INR to guide further therapy. If vitamin K is used to reverse anticoagulation, doses >2 mg can make postoperative reinitiation of anticoagulation more difficult.

The present patient had his warfarin (Coumadin) stopped 5 days before surgery. When his INR was < 2.5, he was started on a full dose of low-molecular-weight heparin. He received the last dose 12 hours before surgery. The patient was restarted on the low-molecular weight heparin and his warfarin at his usual dose 24 hours postoperatively. When the INR was 2.5 for 3 days, the heparin was stopped. The patient had no untoward thromboembolic or bleeding events perioperatively.

Clinical Pearls

1. Patients undergoing most types of dental surgery can continue their usual degree of anticoagulation. Tranexamic acid mouthwash (a fibrinolytic inhibitor) can be used to decrease bleeding, as can local pressure or sutures.

2. Many types of ophthalmologic surgery can be performed safely without reversal of anticoagulation (e.g., cataract surgery, vitreoretinal surgery, and trabeculectomy).

3. It is prudent to discuss the nature of the surgery and the management of the anticoagulant with the ophthamologist preoperatively.

REFERENCES

1. Tinker JH, Tarhan S: Discontinuing anticoagulant therapy in surgical patients with cardiac valve prostheses. JAMA 239:738–739, 1978.
2. Cannegieter SC, Rosendaal FR, Briet E: Thromboembolic and bleeding complications in patients with mechanical heart valve prostheses. Circulation 89:635–641, 1994.
3. Kearon C, Hirsh J: Management of anticoagulation before and after surgery. N Engl J Med 336:1506–1510, 1997.
4. ACC/AHA/ESC Guidelines for the management of patients with atrial fibrillation: Executive summary. Circulation 104:2118–2150, 2001.
5. Jacobs LG, Nusbaum N: Perioperative management and reversal of antithrombotic therapy. Clin Geriat Med 17:189–202, 2001.
6. Spandorfer J: The management of anticoagulation before and after procedures. Med Clin North Am 85:1109–1116, 2001.

PATIENT 66

A 78-year-old man with diarrhea after lumbar decompression

A 78-year-old man underwent lumber decompression for spinal stenosis. He received cefazolin as a perioperative antibiotic, which was continued for 48 hours postoperatively. Four days postoperatively, he began to have loose stools. The following day, his symptoms worsened; he had abdominal tenderness and distention, and multiple watery bowel movements. He remained afebrile but had an increase in his WBC.

Physical Examination: Temperature 99.0°F, pulse 98, respirations 18, blood pressure 110/62. HEENT: normal. Lungs: clear. Heart: regular rhythm. Normal S_1 and S_2. Grade 2/6 systolic murmur at the right upper sternal border without radiation. Abdomen: moderate distention and tympany. Hyperactive bowel sounds, diffusely tender.

Laboratory Findings: WBC 18,300/μL, 14% bands, 81% polymorphonuclear neutrophils, 5% lymphocytes, hematocrit 34.2%, platelets 189,000/μL. Sodium 136 mEq/L, chloride 103 mEq/L, potassium 3.6 mEq/L, bicarbonate 22 mEq/L, BUN 30 mg/dL, creatinine 1.9 mg/dL.

Question: What is the most likely cause of the patient's diarrhea?

Answer: *Clostridium difficile.*

Discussion: *C. difficile* is a gram-positive, spore-forming anaerobic bacillus that received its name because it was "the difficult clostridium" to grow. *C. difficile* produces an enterotoxin (toxin A) and a cytotoxin (toxin B). These toxins produce colonic injury by causing a severe inflammatory reaction in the lamina propria. In severe cases, focal ulceration of the colonic mucosa is followed by subsequent exudation of purulent material and necrotic debris. This material then forms *pseudomembranes,* which appear as small yellow or white plaques during colonoscopy. This is referred to as **pseudomembranous colitis,** or **toxic megacolon,** and is the most feared complication. It develops in only 5% of cases but has a death rate of 65%.

Studies have shown that in addition to antibiotic use, risk factors for *C. difficile* infection include older age, severity of underlying disease, presence of a nasogastric tube, antacid medications, intensive care unit stay, and longer length of hospital stay. Many patients become colonized by *C. difficile,* however, and do not become actively ill. One study showed that serum IgG levels against *C. difficile* toxin A were three times higher in asymptomatic carriers than in patients with active infection. Although almost every antibiotic has been associated with the development of *C. difficile* at one time or another, the most frequently implicated have been the cephalosporins, ampicillin, amoxicillin, and clindamycin.

The clinical presentation is most commonly diarrhea (sometimes prolific), abdominal pain (often cramplike in nature), abdominal distention, fever, and leukocytosis. At times, the leukocytosis and accompanying bandemia can be striking. It sometimes can present in an atypical fashion, for example, as fever of unknown origin or as an ileus without significant diarrhea. The diarrhea may contain mucus and occult blood, but visible blood is rare. Toxic megacolon presents with signs on radiograph that include a dilated colon and thumbprinting of the colon wall; there also may be an ileus present with loops of dilated small bowel.

For diagnosis, enzyme immunoassays often are used because they are rapid and specific, but they are not sensitive (63% in some studies). These tests detect the presence of toxin A or B. The gold standard is the tissue culture cytotoxicity assay. It is slower than other methods, requiring incubation for 24 to 48 hours, and the sensitivity is better than immunoassay. Routine stool culture is time-consuming and is not specific for toxin-producing strains of *C. difficile.* A major advantage of routine culture is that it enables strain typing to identify the cause of outbreaks.

The mainstays of therapy are discontinuation of any causative antibiotic and initiation of oral metronidazole. Rarely, metronidazole is not effective, in which case oral vancomycin should be used. For patients who cannot take medications orally, metronidazole can be used intravenously; because it is excreted into bile, it still reaches adequate treatment levels in the colon. For patients on postoperative warfarin (Coumadin), metronidazole can potentiate warfarin's anticoagulant effects. Cholestyramine at a dose of 4 g four times a day for 1 to 2 weeks can bind the *C. difficile* toxin and can be used with antibiotics for patients who relapse or who are slow to respond to initial therapy. Because cholestyramine can bind the treatment antibiotics, they should be given 2 to 3 hours apart from each other. Antidiarrheal agents such as loperamide should be avoided because they can delay clearance of toxin from the colon and are thought to increase the risk of developing toxic megacolon.

The present patient's initial enzyme immunoassay was negative, but he was started empirically on metronidazole because of the strong clinical suspicion of *C. difficile.* He improved significantly over the first 24 hours. He was treated with metronidazole, 250 mg four times a day for 10 days. The fact that he never developed a fever with his infection is typical of elderly patients, who often remain afebrile despite significant infection.

Clinical Pearls

1. Causes of diarrhea in postoperative patients in addition to *C. difficile* infection include tube feedings, hyperosmolar liquid medications that contain sorbitol (i.e., theophylline and cimetidine), and side effects to medications (especially antibiotics).

2. Extracolonic manifestations of *C. difficile* infection can occur, including involvement of the small intestine, reactive arthritis, bacteremia, encephalopathy, cellulitis, and osteomyelitis.

3. Severe cases of *C. difficile* infection can result in toxic megacolon, electrolyte abnormalities, hypoalbuminemia, bowel perforation, and even death, and must be treated aggressively.

REFERENCES

1. Manabe YC, Vinetz JM, Moore RD, et al. *Clostridium difficile* colitis: An efficient clinical approach to diagnosis. Ann Intern Med 123:835–840, 1995.
2. Harbarth S: Antibiotic prophylaxis and the risk of *Clostridium difficile*–associated diarrhea. J Hosp Infect. 48:93–97, 2001.
3. Jacobs A, Barnard D, Fishel R, Gradon JD: Extracolonic manifestations of *Clostridium difficile* infections. Medicine. 80:88–101, 2001.
4. Kyne L, Farrell RJ, Kelly CP: *Clostridium difficile*. Gastroenterol Clin North Am 30:753–777, 2001.

PATIENT 67

A 26-year-old woman with cirrhosis and postoperative increase in abdominal girth

A 26-year-old woman with a history of morbid obesity had severe steatohepatits that progressed to cirrhosis. She underwent a vertical banded gastroplasty in an effort to lose weight and spare her remaining hepatic function. She also had weight-related type 2 diabetes mellitus and hypertension, which she hoped would improve with weight loss. Her preoperative hepatic function was fairly good based on laboratory findings of albumin 3.2 mg/dL, total bilirubin 2.6 mg/dL, international normalized ratio (INR) 1.3, aspartate transaminase (AST) 52 mg/dL, and alanine transaminase (ALT) 60 mg/dL. On postoperative day 2 she developed significant confusion. On postoperative day 4 she complains of diffuse mild abdominal discomfort and is noted to have increased abdominal girth.

Physical Examination: Vital signs: within normal limits. HEENT: pupils equal, round, and reactive. Sclerae mildly icteric. Lungs: clear. Cardiac: regular rate and rhythm. No murmur, rub, or gallop. Abdomen: obese, distended. Abdominal wound with mild serous drainage. Positive shifting dullness. Mild pretibial edema.

Laboratory Findings: WBC 10,200/μL, with normal differential. Hematocrit 34%. Electrolytes, BUN, creatinine all normal. Ammonia 81 mg/dL, total bilirubin 3.2 mg/dL. AST 70 mg/dL, ALT 72 mg/dL, INR 1.6. Abdominal ultrasound: moderate ascites present.

Question: What caused this patient's confusion?

Diagnosis: Postoperative hepatic encephalopathy.

Discussion: Patients with cirrhosis have increased morbidity and mortality when undergoing major surgery. Many factors contribute. Inhalation anesthetics decrease hepatic blood flow, which can contribute to hepatic ischemia. Hypotension, vasopressors, and hypoxemia also can lead to hepatic ischemia. Although this hepatic ischemia is not generally clinically apparent in patients with healthy livers, it can lead to worsened hepatic function in patients with cirrhosis. Anesthetic agents also can cause direct liver injury; halothane is a classic example. When severe hepatic disease is present, medications such as narcotics or sedatives may have a longer duration of action, with a resultant prolonged decreased level of consciousness, and even can precipitate hepatic encephalopathy.

The most common causes of perioperative mortality are hepatic failure, sepsis, hemorrhage, and the hepatorenal syndrome. Ziser et al[5] found in a retrospective review that the perioperative morbidity rate for patients with cirrhosis was 30.1%, and the mortality rate was 11.6%.

For preoperative risk assessment of patients with chronic liver disease, the Childs classification has been used. Although it originally was devised to provide risk assessment for portocaval shunting, it has been generalized successfully to other types of surgery (see table). Various retrospective studies have found mortality rates in the range of 0 to 10% for class A, 10% to 30% for class B, and 53% to 82% for class C. An updated version of this classification system is the Child-Pugh classification. The major change is that INR substitutes for nutritional status.

In preparing a cirrhotic patient for surgery, several steps should be taken. First, any coagulopathy should be corrected. Vitamin K can be given every day for 3 days in an effort to normalize an increased INR. If vitamin K administration has no significant effect, fresh frozen plasma will be needed perioperatively. Platelet transfusion should be considered to keep the platelet count >50,000/μL for minor surgery, and as close to 100,000/μL as possible for major surgery. If the bleeding time is prolonged significantly, desmopressin can be tried. Electrolyte abnormalities should be corrected, and nutrition should be optimized. If necessary, paracentesis can be done preoperatively to improve the mechanics of breathing and to normalize the abdominal wall before abdominal surgery to decrease risk of wound dehiscence and abdominal wall herniation. Hepatic encephalopathy should be optimized preoperatively as well. Coexisting conditions that can precipitate or worsen encephalopathy include alkalosis, constipation, infection, hypoxia, azotemia, hypokalemia, and gastrointestinal bleeding, and all should be treated as appropriate.

Appropriate anesthetic agents for patients with liver disease include isoflurane, which undergoes only 0.2% hepatic metabolism and may allow increased hepatic arterial blood flow; atracurium, which does not undergo hepatic metabolism, and fentanyl or sufentanil. The best benzodiazepines are oxazepam and lorazepam, which are eliminated by glucuronidation without significant hepatic metabolism.

The present patient was treated with lactulose for new hepatic encephalopathy and received a low-salt diet, spironolactone , and low-dose furosemide for new ascites. The diuretics adequately relieved her ascites so that she did not develop wound dehiscence. Her encephalopathy improved significantly after 5 days, but her ascites persisted for 4 weeks.

Childs Criteria for Assessing Degree of Operative Risk

	Class A	Class B	Class C
Serum bilirubin (mg/dL)	<2.0	2.0–3.0	>3.0
Serum albumin (g/dL)	>3.5	3.0–3.5	<3.0
Ascites	None	Easily	Poorly
Neurologic status/encephalopathy	None	Minimal	Advanced
Nutrition	Excellent	Good	Poor

Clinical Pearls

1. Acute hepatitis, both viral and alcoholic, is a contraindication for elective surgery. The perioperative mortality rate for patients with acute alcoholic hepatitis has been 55%.

2. The perioperative mortality of resection of hepatocellular carcinoma is 3% to 16%.

3. Patients with severe hepatic disease are more susceptible to infection, likely as a result of decreased cell-mediated immunity.

4. Patients with chronic hepatitis who have not progressed to cirrhosis are not at significant perioperative risk.

REFERENCES

1. Pugh RN, Murray-Lyon IM, Dawson JL, et al: Transection of the oesophagus for bleeding oesophageal varices. BMJ 60:646–649, 1973.
2. Gitlin N: Liver disease. In: Lubin MF, Walker HK, Smith RB (eds): Medical Management of the Surgical Patient, 3rd ed. Philadelphia, JB Lipincott, 1995, pp 165–175.
3. Friedman LS: The risk of surgery in patients with liver disease. Hepatology 29:1617–1623, 1999.
4. Patel T. Surgery in the patient with liver disease. Mayo Clin Proc. 74:593–599, 1999.
5. Ziser A, Plevak DJ, Wiesner RH, et al: Morbidity and mortality in cirrhotic patients undergoing anesthesia and surgery. Anesthesiology 90:42–53, 1999.

PATIENT 68

A 60-year-old woman with abdominal distention and nausea after surgery

A 60-year-old woman underwent repair of a cystourethrocele and uterine prolapse. Her medical problems include hypertension, type 2 diabetes mellitus, and hypothyroidism. Her medications postoperatively are oxycodone, diltiazem, NPH insulin, and levothyroxine. Two days postoperatively, she developed mild abdominal distention and nausea. Over the next 2 days, her distention worsens as does her nausea. She has had no bowel movements since 2 days preoperatively and is passing very little flatus.

Physical Examination: Temperature 98.8°F, pulse 80, blood pressure 154/94. Lungs: clear. Heart: normal. Abdomen: significant distention. Tympanic; diffuse mild-to-moderate tenderness on palpation with voluntary guarding. No rebound. Hypoactive bowel sounds. Abdominal radiograph: moderate distention of the large bowel and the small bowel loops. No air-fluid levels.

Laboratory Findings: WBC 9,200/μL, hematocrit 36.6%, platelets 197,000/μL. Sodium 136 mEq/L, potassium 3.2 mEq/L, chloride 101 mEq/L, bicarbonate 27 mEq/L, glucose 210 mg/dL. Liver function tests normal.

Question: What is a major cause of postoperative abdominal distention and discomfort?

Diagnosis: Postoperative ileus.

Discussion: Neuromuscular dysfunction of the bowel is termed **adynamic ileus** and is common in the postoperative setting. Abdominal distention is the most common sign; other common signs and symptoms include nausea, vomiting, mild-to-moderate abdominal pain, tenderness on physical examination, decreased bowel sounds, and decreased stool production. Abdominal radiographs are the most helpful diagnostic tool; patients with a significant ileus may have distended loops of small bowel, a distended colon, and a distended stomach. Adynamic ileus often must be differentiated from a mechanical obstruction, such as a small bowel obstruction or a large bowel obstruction. Small bowel obstruction typically presents on radiograph as air-fluid levels in a stair-step pattern associated with only a small amount of gas in the colon. Obstruction of the colon with a competent ileocecal valve appears on radiograph as gaseous distention confined to the colon; if the ileocecal valve is incompetent, however, gas is present in the small and the large bowel.

A variety of clinical entities have been implicated in the development of paralytic ileus; in many patients, more than one factor is responsible. Postoperative ileus is fairly common, especially in patients who have had surgery within the abdominal cavity. A major factor is thought to be a dysfunction of the enteric nervous system, although this is not well understood. Also important are the effects of medications, especially narcotics and anticholinergic agents, and electrolyte abnormalities.

The mainstays of treatment are reversal of any underlying causes, discontinuation of offending medications, and movement of the patient (e.g., turning a bed-bound patient every 2 hours). A nasogastric tube for decompression of the stomach and small bowel sometimes is necessary as well. If a severe pseudo-obstruction of the colon is present with cecum dilation of >10 cm, consideration should be given to decompression by rectal tube to avoid colonic perforation. In refractory cases, decompression by colonoscopy has been successful.

The present patient required nasogastric decompression for 1 day, which helped relieve the distention, nausea, and vomiting. Her narcotics were held, and her postoperative pain medication was changed to ketorolac (Toradol). She was started on metoclopramide (Reglan) intravenously every 6 hours. Because she had long-standing diabetes, it was unclear whether or not an element of diabetic gastroparesis and intestinal dysmotility also may have played a role. She also was moderately hypokalemic, which likely contributed; she received potassium repletion. Her thyroid-stimulating hormone was checked to ensure that she did not have an element of hypothyroidism. The patient was repositioned frequently and was encouraged to ambulate. Her ileus resolved after 4 days.

Clinical Pearls

1. There are multiple causes of ileus, including spinal cord injury, pancreatitis, peritonitis, the postoperative state, hypokalemia, hypothyroidism, drugs, and systemic illness.

2. Patients with ileus or bowel obstruction often have significant fluid deficits which should be treated.

3. Patients with unusual causes of ileus (i.e., scleroderma or idiopathic pseudo-obstruction) may need more intensive therapy: octreotide given 300–600 μg daily SC in divided doses can be tried.

REFERENCES
1. Dubois A, et al: Postoperative ileus: Physiopathology, etiology, and treatment. Ann Surg 178:781, 1973.
2. Squire LF: Fundamentals of Radiology. Cambridge, MA, Harvard University Press, 1994, pp 168–175.
3. Liolios A, Oropello JM, Benjamin E: Gastrointestinal complications in the intensive care unit. Clin Chest Med 20:329–344, 1999.
4. Sheth SG, LaMont JT: Gastrointestinal problems in the chronically critically ill patient. Clin Chest Med 22:135–147, 2001.

PATIENT 69

A 62-year-old man with hereditary angioneurotic edema anticipating mastoidectomy

A 62-year-old man with hereditary angioneurotic edema (HAE) is referred for evaluation before right mastoidectomy for subacute mastoiditis. For the past 2 months, he has had a "draining ear" unrelieved by oral antibiotics. He recently has developed a facial nerve palsy. CT scan shows extensive involvement of his right mastoid air cells. He has had many episodes of HAE in his lifetime, including some with dyspnea, but has never been intubated. His episodes have been infrequent on stanozolol, 2 mg orally every morning. He has not had an episode in the past 4 years. His mother died at age 65 of HAE, his brother and sister both have HAE, as do one of his two sons and his daughter. He was diagnosed with chronic lymphocytic leukemia 6 years ago. He was treated with chlorambucil and has been in remission up to and including his most recent visit to his oncologist 3 months ago. His influenza and pneumococcal vaccinations are up to date.

Physical Examination: Temperature 98.1°F, pulse 80 and regular, respirations 20, blood pressure 152/90. Skin: warm and moist with a collar of skin tags but no ecchymoses, petechiae, or purpura. HEENT: packing obscuring right ear canal. Lungs: clear to auscultation. Heart: regular without murmurs or gallops. Abdomen: overweight; a firm, nontender, spleen tip descending 4 cm below right rib margin with inhalation. Extremities: no edema. Neuromuscular: right eyelid not blinking, although he is able to close it, but not tightly; no other focal or general deficits.

Laboratory Findings: WBC 48,600/μL, machine differential count 80% granulocytes, hemoglobin 12.7 g/dL, mean corpuscular volume 79 fL, platelets 136,000/μL. Blood chemistries: normal.

Question: What are the patient's risks for perioperative complication?

Answer: Despite the fact that he is improved on stanozolol, he still has episodes, and is at moderate risk for recurrence due to the physiologic stress of surgery.

Discussion: HEA, also known as **hereditary angioedema** and **C1-esterase inhibitor deficiency,** is an autosomal dominant disorder caused by deficiency of the major inhibitor of complement component 1 (C1). This deficiency results in excessive activation of the complement cascade and of kinin-forming cascades, causing acute, severe, focal postcapillary leak with subsequent edema. HAE is characterized by recurrent episodes of nonpruritic edema of the skin, of the gastrointestinal tract, and of the upper respiratory tract, without urticaria. These episodes can be spontaneous and can be induced by minor trauma, surgery, pregnancy, sudden temperature changes, emotional stress, and treatment with angiotension-converting enzyme inhibitors. Attacks occur intermittently throughout life. Gastrointestinal attacks last 1 to 2 days; are self-limited; and consist of vomiting and severe abdominal pain without fever, leukocytosis, or abdominal rigidity. The life-threatening complication is laryngeal edema, which can cause airway obstruction and respiratory failure. Acute episodes have been treated with epinephrine and antifibrinolytic agent ε-aminocaproic acid, fresh frozen plasma, and purified C1-esterase inhibitor, which currently is not available in the United States. Daily use of anabolic steroids can decrease the frequency and severity of the attacks because they increase hepatic synthesis of C1 esterase inhibitor. A condition similar to HAE can be acquired with the formation of antibodies against the C1-esterase inhibitor in patients with lymphoma and other autoimmune disorders.

Because of the present patient's HEA, the clinician must be sure that he is not treated with an angiotension-converting enzyme inhibitor. Throughout the perioperative period, in case he develops evidence of HEA, fresh frozen plasma should be available to transfuse to provide functional C1-esterase inhibitor. If he develops symptomatic laryngeal edema, endotracheal intubation or tracheotomy is the treatment. For patients with severe, frequent, or recent HAE attacks or patients undergoing more extensive surgery, it might be appropriate to provide prophylactic treatment with fresh frozen plasma before surgery. This approach has been used successfully in patients requiring cardiopulmonary bypass. When used prophylactically, fresh frozen plasma can be given as 2 to 4 U within 24 hours preoperatively. The beneficial effect should last 1 to 4 days, after which the C1-esterase inhibitor level returns to its preoperative level. Some clinicians instead have used C1-esterase inhibitor concentrate, which comes with no associated risk of hepatitis. It has been argued that fresh frozen plasma, because it contains complement C2 and C4, theoretically can worsen attacks, but this has not been proved clinically.

The patient's chronic lymphocytic leukemia has returned. His white blood cell count is 48,000/μL, and manual differential revealed the expected abnormal lymphocytes. Although this situation increases his risk for perioperative infectious complications, the planned surgery is indicated to drain the infected mastoid spaces because he has not responded to antibiotic treatment and has developed a cranial nerve palsy. His mild thrombocytopenia is likely due to chronic lymphocyte leukemia; however, he does not have evidence of abnormal hemostasis by history or physical examination, so additional testing and special treatment are not indicated.

The patient's microcytic anemia most likely is due to malabsorption of iron resulting from stanozolol. Intravenous iron treatment might be appropriate after surgery but probably should not be done in the immediate perioperative period because the treatment can increase temporarily the patient's risk for bacteremia.

The patient underwent right mastoidectomy, which cured his infection, without complication.

Clinical Pearls

1. Patients with stable HAE usually can undergo minor procedures without special treatment.

2. Patients with HAE should not be treated with angiotensin-converting enzyme inhibitors becauase these drugs can precipitate attacks.

3. Throughout the perioperative period, the clinician should have fresh frozen plasma ready to transfuse to provide functional C1-esterase inhibitor in case signs or symptoms of an attack of HAE develop.

4. For patients with severe, recent, or frequent HAE attacks or patients undergoing more extensive surgery, it might be appropriate to provide prophylactic treatment with fresh frozen plasma before surgery.

REFERENCES

1. Gadek JE, Hosea SW, Gelfand JA, et al: Replacement therapy in hereditary angioedema: Successful treatment of acute episodes of angioedema with partly purified C1 inhibitor. N Engl J Med 302:542–546, 1980.
2. Wilbur H, Taylor RJ: Prostatectomy in patients with leukemia. Urology, 18:580–581, 1981.
3. Ghosh P, Carroll I, Kanhere A, et al: Cardiac operations in patients with low-grade small lymphocytic malignancies. J Thorac Cardiovasc Surg 118:1033–1037, 1999.
4. Alvarez JM: Successful use of C1 esterase inhibitor protein in a patient with hereditary angioneurotic edema requiring coronary artery bypass surgery. J Thorac Cardiovasc Surg 119:168–171, 2000.
5. Caliezi C, Wuillemin WA, Zeerleder S, et al: C1-Esterase inhibitor: An anti-inflammatory agent and it potential use in the treatment of diseases other than hereditary angioedema. Pharmacol Rev 52:91–112, 2000.
6. Sarantopoulos CD, Brantanow NC, Stowe DF, Kampine JP: Uneventful propofol anesthesia in a patient with co-existing hereditary coproporphyria and hereditary angioneurotic edema. Anesthesiology 92:607–609, 2000.

PATIENT 70

A 19-year-old woman with cyanotic heart disease anticipating wisdom teeth extraction

A 19-year-old woman with cyanotic heart disease is referred for evaluation before having four wisdom teeth extracted. She is a high school senior, living with her mother. She reports having heart surgery as a child and also 5 years previously, and an irregular heartbeat that is controlled with medication. Her medications are atenolol, 25 mg; enalapril, 5 mg; and penicillin 250 mg, all taken twice a day.

Physical Examination: Temperature 97.7°F; pulse regular, 68; respirations 16; blood pressure 90/72. Skin: no lesions; nails cyanotic (Figure). HEENT: lips cyanotic (Figure), otherwise normal. Chest: median sternotomy scar, clear to auscultation. Heart: apical impulse 4 cm in diameter, 5 cm from midsternal line in fifth intercostal space, S_4 at apex, no murmurs. Abdomen: normal. Extremities: clubbing (bottom Figure). Neuromuscular: normal.

Question: What should be done to prepare her for dental extractions?

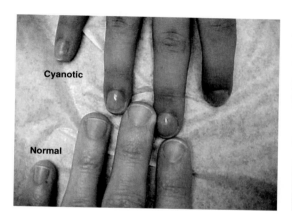

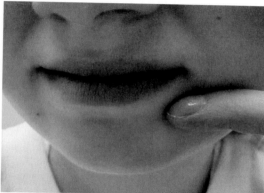

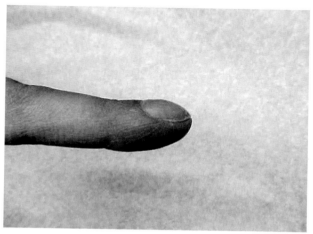

Answer: (1) Obtain her prior medical records; (2) ensure that she is not pregnant; (3) assess her functional capacity; (4) obtain baseline oximetry; (5) advise her on perioperative medication management; (6) arrange for endocarditis prophylaxis; (7) review her primary care needs.

Discussion: A thorough medication history is crucial to good perioperative care, and obtaining one often requires specific prompting. It also is crucial to determine whether a woman of child-bearing age is pregnant before proceeding to anesthesia and surgery. Strong consideration should be given to checking a serum or urine pregnancy test in all women of child-bearing age, regardless of contraceptives, because no form of birth control except abstinence is absolute. Likewise, assessing functional capacity is important. In a reliable patient, a questionnaire usually is all that is needed to assess functional capacity. There are several validated questionnaires for assessing functional capacity (e.g., see the Duke Functional Activity Scale[1]). If functional capacity is poor or has declined recently, additional testing may be appropriate.

It was suspected the present patient was also taking anticoagulant medication for her heart disease. On specific questioning, she reported 1 baby aspirin (81 mg) daily. Because she was of child-bearing age, she was explicitly asked about birth control, and she reported receiving medroxyprogesterone (Depo-Provera), 150 mg intramuscularly every 3 months. From her cardiologist's office a more detailed medical and surgical history was obtained as follows:

Corrected transposition of the great arteries, atrial septal defect, large ventricular septal defect, and tricuspid atresia. Surgical repairs at age 3, 13, and 15. She discontinued warfarin 1 year ago at age 18.
Paroxysmal supraventricular tachycardia controlled on atenolol.
Congenital asplenia for which she takes daily penicllin prophylaxis against pneumococcal and streptococcal infections.

Routine testing 4 months previously showed the following:

ECG: normal sinus rhythm 60, a surgical loop axis with inverted P waves in lead I, right ventricular hypertrophy with upright T waves in V1, deep S across precordium, and nonspecifically abnormal T waves and ST segments.
Echocardiography: prior Fontan operation, with patent lateral tunnel, no tunnel-arterial shunt, trivial atrioventricular valve regurgitation, and globally reduced ventricular wall motion.
24-hour Holter monitor: rare isolated premature ventricular contractions.

To assess her functional capacity, the patient was asked several specific questions. She reported that she could carry 10 kg up two floors nonstop (7–10 METS) and that she had no dyspnea walking up to a half mile at a normal pace on level ground. With a hand-held oximeter, it was determined that her baseline arterial oxygen saturation was 80%, at rest and after 2 minutes of brisk walking.

Although no additional laboratory testing is indicated in this patient, it is important to obtain a copy of her previous ECG to serve as a baseline in the perioperative period. Similarly, because she is cyanotic, her arterial oxygen saturation will be abnormal. Determining her baseline arterial oxygen saturation can be helpful in her perioperative management. In addition, it is important to state in the report that her systemic blood pressure is deliberately kept low (systolic 90 mmHg) to minimize pulmonary hypertension that results because she has a single heart ventricle supplying systemic and pulmonary circulations. This information will help to guide her perioperative management.

The patient should receive prophylaxis against bacterial endocarditis (see table). She was prescribed clindamycin, 600 mg, to take orally 1 hour before dental work. Amoxicillin and ampicillin are likely to be less effective because her daily

Patient Risk for Endocarditis

High risk:
  Prosthetic valve, including bioprosthetic
  Prior bacterial endocarditis
  Complex cyanotic heart disease
  Surgically constructed systemic pulmonary
    shunts or conduits
Moderate risk:
  Acquired valve disease (e.g., rheumatic)
  Hypertrophic cardiomyopathy
  Mitral valve prolapse with thickened leaflets
    or regurgitation
  Other, not explicitly high or negligible risk
Negligible risk:
  Isolated Secundum ASD
  Surgically repaired ASD, VSD, or PDA ($>$ 6
    months post repair)
  Prior CABG surgery
  Mitral valve prolapse without thickened
    leaflets or regurgitation
  Murmur without an at-risk condition
  Prior Kawasaki's disease or rheumatic fever
    without valve dysfunction
  Cardiac pacers, even intravascular

ASD, atrial septal defect, VSD, ventricular septal defect; PDA, patent ductus arteriosus; CABG, coronary artery bypass graft.

penicillin treatment has led to her mouth being colonized with penicillin-resistant bacteria. There are several alternative antibiotics for endocarditis prophylaxis (see table).

In addition, because of the prevalence of penicillin-resistant pneumococcus, the patient was not receiving adequate prophylaxis against pneumococcal infections. She should receive the pneumococcal vaccine, and, possibly, the more immunogenic conjugated pneumococcal vaccine. She should receive the meningococcal vaccine if she enters a high-risk situation, such as her first year living at college. Finally, she should receive influenza vaccination annually.

To minimize bleeding, the patient was advised to stop her daily aspirin 7 days before dental extractions and to resume aspirin the day after dental work. Managing anticoagulation in patients at risk for pathologic thrombosis in the perioperative period is not strictly formulaic but requires individualizing recommendations in an attempt to balance the risks of pathologic thrombosis with beneficial clotting. She also was advised to continue her medications on the day of dental work. Because she is asplenic, the pneumococcal vaccine was administered, and the patient was advised to have it boosted every 6 years and to obtain the influenza vaccine annually. She subsequently underwent extraction of four molars without complication.

Antibiotics for Prophylaxis Against Endocarditis

Dental and upper respiratory procedures
Orally, 1 hour before procedure
  Amoxicillin, 2 g, or clindamycin, 600 mg, or cephalexin, 2 g, or clarithromycin, 500 mg, or azithromycin, 500 mg
Intravenously, 1 hour before procedure
  Ampicillin, 2 g, or clindamycin 600 mg, or cefazolin, 1 g
Gastrointestinal and genitourinary procedures
Orally, 1 hour before the procedure
  Amoxicillin 2 gm
Intravenously, 1 hour before the procedure
  Ampicillin, 2 g, or vancomycin, 1 g
  High-risk patients also should receive gentamicin, 1.5 mg/kg (up to 120 mg)

Clinical Pearls

1. Obtaining a thorough medication history often requires specific prompting.
2. Ascertain whether a woman of child-bearing age is pregnant before proceeding to surgery.
3. A specific questionnaire usually is all that is needed to assess functional capacity.
4. Patients at risk for bacterial endocarditis should receive appropriate prophylaxis.

REFERENCES

1. Hlatky MA, Boineau RE, Higginbotham MB, et al: A brief self-administered questionnaire to determine functional capacity (the Duke Activity Status Index). Am J Cardiol 64:651–654, 1989.
2. Dajani AS, Taubert KA, Wilson W, et al: Prevention of bacterial endocarditis: Recommendations by the American Heart Association. JAMA 277:1794–1801, 1997.
3. Pierre N, Moy LK, Redd S, et al: Evaluation of a pregnancy-testing protocol in adolescents undergoing surgery. J Pediatr Adolesc Gynecol 11:139–141, 1998.
4. Reilly DF, McNeely MJ, Doerner D, et al: Self-reported exercise tolerance and the risk of serious perioperative complications. Arch Intern Med 159:2185–2192, 1999.
5. Lau HS, Florax C, Porsius AJ, De Boer A: The completeness of medication histories in hospital medical records of patients admitted to general internal medicine wards. Br J Clin Pharmacol 49:597–603, 2000.

PATIENT 71

A 68-year-old woman with fatigue anticipating cholecystectomy

A 68-year-old woman is referred for evaluation before cholecystectomy. For the past 6 months, she has had progressive fatigue, weakness, and abdominal pain. To evaluate her fatigue, she underwent complete cardiac and pulmonary evaluations, but these were unrevealing. Transthoracic echocardiography showed a left ventricular ejection fraction of 68%, mild aortic insufficiency and sclerosis without stenosis, and mild atherosclerosis of the descending aorta. Spirometry showed mild overinflation with air trapping. High-resolution CT scan of the chest showed only small patches of atelectasis without fibrosis. Pulmonary exercise testing showed a good heart rate and ventilatory reserve but severe exercise impairment with a markedly reduced anaerobic threshold and an increased ventilatory requirement of "undiscerned cause." To evaluate her abdominal pain, she underwent colonoscopy, which showed only diverticulosis, and abdominal CT, which showed only cholelithiasis. Cholecystectomy was scheduled. Her surgeon thinks that her symptoms are not due to cholelithiasis and requests a preoperative medical evaluation. Her medical history includes mild hypertension, treated with triamterene and hydrochlorothiazide, and hypothyroidism resulting from thyroidectomy for thyroid cancer 35 years ago, treated with levothyroxine. She received radioactive iodine treatment 10 years ago for locally recurrent thyroid cancer. She continues to swim 1 mile daily but now is unable to pull herself out of the pool.

Physical Examination: Temperature 99.0°F; pulse regular, seated 98, supine 68; respirations 14; Blood pressure seated 100/70. Skin: warm, dry with faint yellowish "suntan" over entire body and faint pigmentation of palmar creases, no axillary hair, sparse head and pubic hair, capillary fragility ecchymoses on forearms. HEENT: horizontal surgical scar low on anterior neck, no palpable thyroid or adenopathy, normal carotid upstrokes. Lungs: clear to auscultation. Heart: regular rhythm with III/VI systolic murmur heard best with bell at right second intercostal space radiating to neck. Abdomen: benign. Extremities: no edema. Neuromuscular: alert, oriented, appropriate, cranial nerves II through XII grossly intact, strength 5/5 symmetric, sensation intact to light touch, slight irregular tremor of extended limbs, mild symmetric hyperreflexia with nonsustained clonus, gait normal.

Laboratory Findings: CBC and blood chemistries normal. Ionized calcium: normal. Serum liver tests: normal. Thyroid-stimulating hormone: low normal. ECG: normal. Chest radiograph: trace left lower lobe atelectasis.

Questions: What is causing this woman's abdominal pain? Should she undergo cholecystectomy?

Answer: Primary corticoadrenal insufficiency, confirmed by a low plasma cortisol and an elevated ACTH.

Discussion: This patient's illness was diagnosed by history and physical examination after many sophisticated and expensive tests and imaging studies were unrevealing. Had she proceeded to surgery, she would have been at greater than usual risk for postoperative complication, and she might have suffered cardiovascular collapse. The symptoms of adrenal insufficiency, such as weakness, fatigue, nausea, and abdominal pain, are nonspecific; however, this patient's physical findings, including hyperpigmentation, hypotrichosis, and orthostatic hypotension made the diagnosis apparent.

Endogenous glucocorticoids produced in the adrenal glands are necessary for life. Glucocorticoid receptors are found in all cells. They are required for normal cellular metabolism and homeostasis. Glucocorticoids are produced in, and released from the adrenal glands in response to adrenocorticotropic hormone (ACTH) from the pituitary, which is, in turn produced and released in response to stimulation by corticotropin-releasing hormone (CRH) from the hypothalamus. Cortisol is the main endogenous glucocorticoid.

Endogenous mineralocorticoids are also produced in the adrenal glands. They are necessary for sodium and potassium homeostasis, and to maintain intravascular volume. Aldosterone is the main endogenous mineralocorticoid. Also, in women adrenal androgens are necessary for maintaining axillary and pubic hair, and they contribute significantly to maintenance of muscle mass and sexual drive.

Normal production of endogenous glucocorticoids is estimated to be 5 to 10 mg of cortisol per meter squared of body surface area per day. This is equal to 20 to 30 mg of hydrocortisone or 5 to 7 mg of prednisone per day in a normal adult. Glucocorticoid release varies throughout the day with a large release about 6 AM and minimal release from evening until early morning. Under severe physiologic stress there is a ten-fold increase in the release of endogenous glucocorticoids.

Adrenal insufficiency can be due to a defect in the adrenal gland (primary), in the pituitary (secondary), or in the hypothalamus (tertiary). It can occur acutely or, as in this patient, chronically. Primary adrenal insufficiency is due to destruction of the adrenal glands and is not manifest until at least 90% of the gland is destroyed. Primary adrenal insufficiency is rare, with a prevalence of about 1:10,000 adults in the United States. It is most often (80%) due to autoimmune disease, although the highly vascular adrenal gland can be replaced by tuberculoma, histoplasmoma, or metastatic tumor. In developing countries, tuberculosis is the most common cause of primary adrenal insufficiency. Secondary adrenal insufficiency is uncommon and is caused by pituitary destruction, as from head injury, pituitary hemorrhage and infarction (Sheehan's syndrome), or pituitary tumor. It can be associated with panhypopituitarism, which is insufficiency of other pituitary hormones, such as thyroid-stimulating hormone and growth hormone. In contrast to primary adrenal insufficiency, adrenal mineralocorticoid function is usually intact in secondary adrenal insufficiency. Because the present patient had compromised mineralocorticoid function and a high serum adrenocorticotropic hormone (ACTH) level, her adrenal insufficiency was primary.

The most common type of adrenal insufficiency is tertiary adrenal insufficiency caused by suppression of hypothalamic corticotropin-releasing hormone secretion by treatment with exogenous corticosteroid. In a patient with suspected adrenal insufficiency, it is important to ascertain prior steroid use. The hypothalamic-pituitary-adrenal axis can be suppressed for 1 year after exogenous corticosteroid treatment.

Testing for adrenal insufficiency can start with determination of 8 A.M. plasma cortisol and ACTH. If cortisol is <5 μg/dL (140 nmol/L), the patient is adrenally insufficient, and if it is >20 μg/dL (550 nmol/L), the patient is not adrenally insufficient. If the patient is adrenally insufficient and the ACTH concentration is >150 pg/mL (22 pmol/L), the patient has primary adrenal insufficiency. If the ACTH concentration is lower, the patient has secondary or tertiary adrenal insufficiency. The difficulty in diagnosis occurs in patients with intermediate cortisol concentrations. A corticotropin stimulation test (CST) can exclude primary adrenal insufficiency. A CST consists of the administration of 250 μg of corticotropin (cosyntropin) intravenously or intramuscularly in the morning before 10 A.M. The plasma cortisol is measured before, and 30 and 60 minutes after injection of corticotropin. A cortisol concentration >20 μg/dL at any time rules out primary adrenal insufficiency. Mild secondary or tertiary adrenal insufficiency still might be present. Prolonged secondary or tertiary adrenal insufficiency can lead to adrenal atrophy, making the adrenal glands unable to respond to the CST. If secondary or tertiary adrenal insufficiency still is suspected in patients with a normal response to the CST, head MRI should be considered to rule out pituitary or hypothalamic mass lesions. In patients with indeterminate results, a test for serum antibodies to 21-hydroxylase can rule out primary autoimmune adrenal insufficiency. Such antibodies are present in virtually all patients with autoimmune adrenalitis of <10 years' duration. Finally, adrenal CT or MRI can rule out adrenal atrophy or mass lesions.

The present patient was given adrenal replacement doses of hydrocortisone, her diuretic was discontinued, and her symptoms resolved. Surgery was cancelled. Abdominal CT showed small adrenal glands without masses or calcification. After a few months, she also required fludrocortisone mineralocorticoid replacement.

Clinical Pearls

1. A thoughtful general medical evaluation can be of value in patients with confusing symptoms before surgery.
2. Adrenal insufficiency resulting from prior steroid use is the most common type of adrenal insufficiency in the developed world.

REFERENCES
1. Jabbour SA: Steroids and the surgical patient. Med Clin North Am 85:1311–1317, 2001.
2. Ten S, New M, Maclaren N: Clinical review 130: Addison's disease. J Clin Endocrinol Metab 86:2090–2122, 2001.
3. Coursin DB, Wood KE: Corticosteroid supplementation for adrenal insufficiency. JAMA 287:236–240, 2002.

PATIENT 72

A 32-year-old woman with a renal transplant anticipating hysterectomy

A 32-year-old woman is referred for evaluation before hysterectomy for dysfunctional uterine bleeding. Ten years ago, she developed nephrotic syndrome secondary to idiopathic glomerular sclerosis, for which she was treated with prednisone. Five years ago, she began hemodialysis, and 3 years ago, she received a cadaveric renal transplant with subsequent good renal function. Before the transplant, she was amenorrheic, but afterward she gradually developed dysfunctional uterine bleeding unresponsive to estrogen suppression. She also recently developed severe dyspareunia. Her gynecologist advises hysterectomy and requests preoperative evaluation and recommendations for perioperative care. Her current medications are atorvastatin (Lipitor), 10 mg orally daily; lisinopril (Prinivil), 2.5 orally daily; amlodipine (Norvasc), 5 mg orally daily; atenolol, 50 mg orally daily; furosemide, 40 mg orally daily; cyclosporine (Neoral), 150 mg orally twice a day; mycophenolate mofetil (CellCept), 1,000 mg orally twice a day; prednisone, 10 mg orally daily; and trimethoprim-sulfamethoxazole (Bactrim DS), 160 to 800 mg orally every Monday, Wednesday, and Friday. She reports jogging 3 miles twice a week.

Physical Examination: Temperature 98.1°F; pulse regular 68, respirations 14, blood pressure 120/82. Height 66 inches, weight 142 lb. General appearance: Cushingoid. Skin: warm and dry without ecchymoses. HEENT: normal. Lungs: clear to auscultation. Heart: regular without murmurs or gallops. Abdomen: soft, nontender, without hepatosplenomegaly. Extremities: no edema. Neuromuscular: no gross deficits.

Laboratory Findings: WBC 7,000/μL, hemoglobin 11.1 g/dL. Serum electrolytes normal. Serum creatinine 1.5 mg/dL. Cyclosporine 12-hour trough by high-performance liquid chromatography 156 (therapeutic range in first year after transplant 200 to 400, after first year 100 to 200). ECG: normal.

Question: What are the patient's risks for perioperative complication?

Answer: Risks include development of fluid overload, hyponatremia, hyperkalemia, and acute renal failure.

Discussion: Perioperative risks faced by patients with a renal transplant can be separated into those due to a low glomerular filtration rate (GRF) and those due to immunosuppressive medications. A low GFR increases the risk for perioperative complications resulting from fluid overload. Because anesthesia and surgery induce generalized vasodilation, additional intravascular fluid is needed to maintain blood pressure and tissue perfusion. This need is met by intravenous infusion of fluid. As the patient recovers from surgery and the vasodilation resolves, the additional fluid must be excreted. Because of the low GFR, water and solutes cannot be excreted rapidly, and there can be a period when the vasodilation has resolved but the additional fluid remains. This excess fluid can lead to an overexpanded intravascular volume causing hypertension and, in some patients, pulmonary edema.

A low GFR also increases the risk for perioperative hyponatremia. The low GFR diminishes the ability of the kidney to generate dilute urine. This problem is exacerbated in the perioperative period by the release of antidiuretic hormone caused by stimuli such as trauma, pain, nausea, and perioperative medications such as opiates. It can be exacerbated further by the infusion of hyponatremic fluids, such as 0.45 normal saline. There is evidence that premenopausal women, such as the present patient, are particularly susceptible to developing hyponatremia in the perioperative period. A low GFR also increases the risk for perioperative hyperkalemia by reducing the ability of the kidney to excrete excess potassium, which can come from medications, intravenous fluids, and cytolysis.

A low GFR increases the risk for perioperative acute renal failure. In the perioperative period, medications, pain, nausea, and blood loss can cause systemic hypotension. Glomerular afferent arteriole vasodilation and efferent arteriole vasoconstriction can increase glomerular blood pressure to compensate for systemic hypotension and to maintain glomerular perfusion. Impairment of this mechanism for regulating glomerular perfusion can reduce an already low GFR to an inadequate GFR, leading to acute renal failure. An acute reduction in glomerular perfusion can cause tubular ischemia, leading to acute tubular necrosis. Medications that impair afferent arteriole vasodilation, such as nonsteroidal antiinflammatory drugs (NSAIDs), and medications that impair efferent arteriole vasoconstriction, such as angiotensin-converting enzyme (ACE) inhibitors, increase the risk of acute renal failure in the perioperative period. Although in the long-term ACE inhibitors preserve renal function by reducing glomerular blood pressure, in the perioperative period they increase the risk for acute renal failure by impairing the kidney's ability to respond to systemic hypotension. Many experts recommend holding ACE inhibitors before surgery.

Patients with a renal transplant are at risk as a result of the effects of immunosuppressive medications, including immunosuppression, hemodynamic and metabolic effects, and medication interactions. Immunosuppression increases the risk for chronic infections caused by bacteria, fungi, viruses and protozoans. Immunosuppressive medications can blunt the manifestations of infection, including elevated WBC and fever. To avoid taking a chronically infected patient to surgery, the preoperative evaluation should include careful assessment for any subtle symptoms or signs of infection. Although patients receiving immunosuppressive medications might be at a higher risk for acute perioperative infections, prophylactic measures are the same as those for nonimmunosuppressed patients.

The hemodynamic and metabolic effects of immunosuppressive medication vary depending on the medication. Cyclosporine (Neoral, Sandimmune) and tacrolimus (Prograf) increase the risk of fluid overload, hyperkalemia, and acute renal failure because they cause afferent arteriole vasoconstriction leading to decreased glomerular perfusion. Although azathioprine (Imuran) and mycophenolate mofetil (CellCept) do not affect glomerular filtration, both are myelosuppressive and can cause leukopenia and thrombocytopenia. In general, immunosuppressive medications adversely affect serum lipids, accelerating atherosclerosis, and should be considered an additional risk factor for ischemic heart disease.

Immunosuppressive medications frequently interact with other medications. Allopurinol inhibits azathioprine metabolism, and the combination can lead to severe myelosuppression. Many hepatically metabolized medications change the rate of metabolism of cyclosporine and can cause subtherapeutic or toxic cyclosporine levels (see table). Cyclosporine also can increase the toxic potential of other medications by inhibiting their hepatic metabolism. Cyclosporine prolongs the effect of fentanyl. Cyclosporine usually should be discontinued in the perioperative period.

Corticosteroid medications should be continued at the patient's usual dose up to the day of surgery. For procedures involving only minor physiologic stress, the patient's usual dose of

Some Cyclosporine-Medication Interactions	
Increase Cyclosporine Level	Decrease Cyclosporine Level
Diltiazem	Penobarbitol
Nicardipine	Phenytoin
Ketoconazole	Carbamazepine
Fluconazole	Trimethoprim-sulfamethoxazole
Ciprofloxacin	
Erythromycin	Rifampin
Clarithromycin	Isoniazid
Cimetidine	
Oral contraceptives	

steroid should be continued throughout the perioperative period; however, for more stressful procedures, supplemental steroid is indicated. Patients taking ≤5 mg/d of prednisone usually do not require steroid supplementation. Patients taking >5 mg/d of prednisone might have suppression of the hypothalamic-pituitary-adrenal axis and should receive supplemental steroid for stressful procedures. If a patient taking ≥5 mg/d of prednisone develops perioperative complications, he or she might benefit from supplemental steroid. For a procedure involving minor stress, such as inguinal herniorrhaphy, a single dose of hydrocortisone hemisuccinate, 25 mg intravenously, or methylprednisolone, 5 mg intravenously, at the start of surgery should be adequate. For a more stressful procedure, such as cholecystectomy or hemicolectomy, hydrocortisone hemisuccinate, 50 mg intravenously every 8 hours, or methylprednisolone, 10 mg intravenously every 6 hours, starting at the time of surgery and tapered over 1 to 2 days should be adequate. For major surgery, such as major cardiothoracic or major abdominal surgery, hydrocortisone hemisuccinate, 100 mg intravenously every 8 hours, or methylprednisolone, 20 mg intravenously every 6 hours, tapered over 2 to 3 days should be adequate.

The present patient did not need additional cardiac evaluation because she had few risk factors for atherosclerotic ischemic heart disease and reported a good functional capacity without symptoms of heart disease. She was advised to:

1. Stop cyclosporine the night prior and day of surgery.
2. Stop lisinopril the day of surgery.
3. Stop any aspirin or NSAIDs for the week before surgery.

Her perioperative caregivers were advised to:

1. Administer hydrocortisone hemisuccinate, 50 mg intravenously every 8 hours, starting at initiation of surgery and tapered to her usual dose over the first postoperative day.
2. Avoid fluid overload and follow closely her serum BUN, creatinine, and electrolytes after surgery.
3. Resume her usual medications when she was able to take them orally.

Her surgery went well, and the patient recovered without complication.

Clinical Pearls

1. Before elective surgery, patients taking immunosuppressive medications should be screened carefully for subtle signs of infection.
2. Patients with tenuous renal function should avoid aspirin and NSAIDs for the week before surgery; the clinician should consider holding ACE inhibitors on the morning of surgery.
3. Cyclosporine should be discontinued the day before surgery and restarted when the patient can resume oral medications.
4. The clinician should check for medication interactions.
5. Fluid overload should be assiduously avoided, and renal function and serum electrolytes should be followed closely after surgery.

REFERENCES
1. Falkenhain ME, Hartman J, Hebert L: Management of water, sodium, potassium, chloride, and magnesium in renal disease and renal failure. In Kopple JD, Massry SG (eds): Nutritional Management of Renal Disease. Baltimore: Williams & Wilkins, 1997.
2. Fishman JA, Rubin RH: Infection in organ-transplant recipients. N Engl J Med 338:1741–1751, 1998.
3. Mueller C, Buerkle G, Buettner HJ, et al: Prevention of contrast media-associated nephropathy: Randomized comparison of 2 hydration regimens in 1620 patients undergoing coronary angioplasty. Arch Intern Med 162:329–336, 2002.
4. Hederman JH: Action, efficacy and toxicities: Cyclosporine. In: Norma DJ, Turka LA (eds): Primer in Transplantation, 2nd ed. Mt. Laurel, NJ, American Society of Transplantation, 2001, p 125.

PATIENT 73

A 66-year-old man with arm deep vein thrombosis 6 days after major head and neck cancer surgery

A 66-year-old man is referred for refractory deep vein thrombosis of the left arm 8 days after resection of stage IV squamous cell carcinoma of the tongue. Six days after surgery, while receiving subcutaneous unfractionated heparin, 5,000 U twice a day; he developed pain, swelling, and ecchymosis of the left hand and forearm. Despite removal of the left subclavian venous catheter, discontinuation of unfractionated heparin, and treatment with subcutaneous dalteparin (Fragmin), 5,000 U twice a day, the left arm pain, swelling, and ecchymosis have progressed.

Physical Examination: Temperature 37.8° C, pulse 88, respirations 18, blood pressure 130/80. Skin: no rash or petechiae, purpura. HEENT: normal postsurgical findings except mild purulent drainage from surgical wound. Chest: clear to auscultation. Heart: regular rhythm without gallops or murmurs. Abdomen: obese, no apparent splenomegaly. Extremities: left arm cool and tender, left hand swollen and ecchymotic with dorsal hemorrhagic bullae, right great toe with distal ecchymosis (Figures). Neuromuscular: no sensation to touch in distal left hand, otherwise normal.

Laboratory Findings: WBC 9,100/μL, granulocytes 78%, hemoglobin 10 g/dL, platelet count: 21,000/μL, preoperative platelet count 268,000/μL. International normalized ratio 1.2. Partial thromboplastin time 32 seconds. Blood chemistries normal. ECG normal. Chest radiograph normal. Doppler ultrasound (6 days after surgery): no flow in left subclavian, axillary, brachial, and basilic veins.

Questions: What is the cause of the patient's deep vein thrombosis? What is the most appropriate treatment?

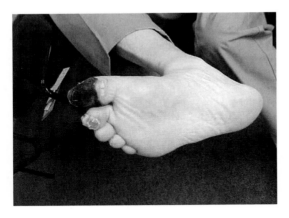 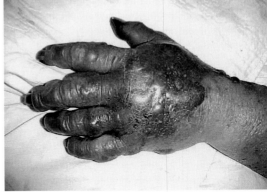

Diagnosis and Treatment: Heparin-induced thrombocytopenia with thrombosis (HITT), complicated by gangrene. Initial therapy should include discontinuation of all heparins, both unfractionated and low-molecular-weight heparins by any route, including heparin flushes and heparin-coated vascular catheters.

Discussion: Acute deep vein thrombosis distal to a venous catheter in a patient after cancer surgery might be caused by decreased velocity of venous return owing to the catheter and thrombophilia owing to the cancer and the surgery. Nonetheless, a broad differential diagnosis should include heparin-induced thrombocytopenia (HIT) and should lead to measuring the platelet count. A system of automatic platelet counts every 3 days for patients receiving heparin might reveal thrombocytopenia before thrombosis is clinically evident.

Thrombocytopenia (a platelet count of <150,000/μL) is caused by decreased platelet production, increased platelet destruction, splenic sequestration of platelets, or a combination of these processes (see Table). To determine the duration of the abnormality, the clinician should review previous medical records and ask the patient about abnormal bleeding after previous surgical or dental procedures. The patient should be examined for evidence of inadequate hemostasis. Petechiae, purpura, and ecchymoses should be sought in locations of the body subject to chronic, mild trauma, such as the buccal mucosa and the soles of the feet. The clinician should carefully

---

Causes of Thrombocytopenia

- Decreased platelet production
  Vitamin B_{12} or folate deficiency
  Drug-induced myelosuppression
  Aplastic anemia
  Leukemia
- Increased platelet destruction
  Heart-lung bypass
  Disseminated intravascular coagulation
  Thrombotic thrombocytopenic purpura
  Pregnancy-induced (hemolysis elevated
    liver enzymes low platelets [HELLP])
  Infection-induced (hemolytic-uremic
    syndrome)
  Drug-induced
  Blood transfusion–induced
  Idiopathic thrombocytopenic purpura
- Splenic sequestration
  Cirrhosis, portal or splenic vein thrombosis
  Lymphomas and leukemias
  Splenic infiltrative diseases (e.g., amyloid,
    Gaucher's)
  Infections (e.g., bacterial endocarditis,
    malaria, visceral leishmaniasis)

---

percuss and palpate for splenomegaly. Overweight patients may require abdominal imaging to assess spleen size adequately. Laboratory examination should include CBC and peripheral blood smear, to assess all blood cell components, platelet size, and evidence of platelet clumping. A small mean platelet volume might be due to many smaller, older platelets because of decreased platelet production, whereas a large mean platelet volume might be due to many large immature platelets because of increased platelet destruction. The clinician should look for pseudothrombocytopenia on the blood smear as platelet clumping caused by the ethylenediaminetetra-acetic acid used to anticoagulate blood specimens. If initial testing is not revealing, bone marrow aspiration might be helpful.

Medications are a common cause of thrombocytopenia in hospitalized patients. Medications can cause myelosuppression (e.g., thiazide diuretics, ticlopidine, ethanol) and can induce an immunologic response (e.g., quinidine, penicillin, heparin). There are two types of heparin-associated thrombocytopenia (HAT). HAT type 1 is caused by the direct binding of heparin to receptors on the platelet surface, which induces platelet activation and destruction. It is dose dependent and is not immune mediated. HAT type 1 occurs in one third of patients who receive heparin, but it rarely causes clinically significant thrombocytopenia.

HAT type 2, or HIT, occurs in 3% to 5% of patients receiving heparin. It usually is noted after 6 to 10 days of heparin administration but can occur more quickly in patients who received heparin in the prior 3 months and can occur a few weeks after heparin is discontinued. Although HIT is usually mild (platelet count >50,000/μL), if heparin is not discontinued the consequences can be catastrophic. HIT is immune mediated and is independent of the dose and route of administration of heparin. As in HAT type 1, heparin binds to the platelet surface, specifically to platelet factor 4 (PF4). In HIT, antibodies are formed against the heparin-PF4 complex causing a conformational change in PF4. The Fc portion of antibody bound to the heparin-PF4 complex also binds to Fc receptors on the platelet surface, which activates the platelet, leading to a cascade of platelet clumping and thrombosis. Thrombotic complications include arterial and venous thrombosis, pulmonary embolism, myocardial infarction, and stroke. As in the present patient, thrombotic complications while on heparin therapy can be misconstrued as treatment failure rather than HITT.

The primary treatment is discontinuation of all heparins, both unfractioned and low-molecular-weight heparins by any route, including heparin flushes and heparin-coated vascular catheters. Although the incidence of HIT as a result of primary use of low-molecular-weight heparins is low, cross-reactivity of low-molecular-weight heparin to HIT-associated IgG is 80% to 100%, and low-molecular-weight heparin use can precipitate catastrophic complications in patients with HIT. Although heparinoids such as danaparoid have been used successfully in small trials, and treatment with intravenous IgG has been helpful in some patients, the principal treatment for thrombotic complications of HIT should be with nonheparin anticoagulants, excluding warfarin. Warfarin is likely to exacerbate the thrombosis by inactivating the anticoagulant protein C more quickly than it inactivates the procoagulant proteins.

Currently the two nonheparin anticoagulants for treating HITT are lepirudan (Refludan) and argatroban. Lepirudan is recombinant hirudan, a direct thrombin inhibitor, officially approved by the U.S. Food and Drug Administration (FDA) for the treatment of HITT in 1998. The usual dose for lepirudin is a 0.4 mg/kg bolus followed by 0.15 mg/kg/h constant infusion adjusted to a target activated partial thromboplastin time (aPTT) 1.5 to 2.5 times control. Dose adjustment is required in patients with renal insufficiency. Argatroban, a synthetic L-arginine derivative, is a reversible direct thrombin inhibitor, approved by the FDA in 2000 for prophylaxis or treatment of thrombosis in patients with HIT. The recommended infusion rate is 0.002 mg/kg/min to achieve a aPTT 1.5 to 3 times control. Dose adjustment is required in patients with significant hepatic impairment. When adequate anticoagulation has been achieved with either lepirudan or argatroban, warfarin can be started for long-term anticoagulation.

Subsequent use of heparin in patients with history of HIT is possible. In many patients with HIT, antibodies against the heparin-PF4 complex are undetectable after 3 months without exposure to heparins. Many of these patients subsequently have undergone surgical procedures using heparin without complication.

The present patient was anticoagulated with lepirudin. Warfarin was added after the target aPTT was achieved. His platelet count returned to baseline, but hand and toe amputation ultimately were required (Figure).

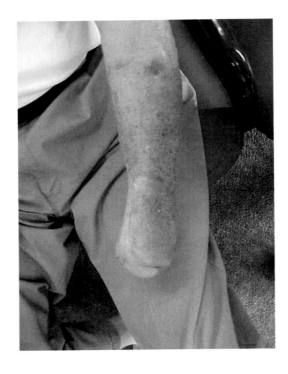

Clinical Pearls

1. Of patients receiving heparin, in any form, 1% to 5% develop heparin antibodies.
2. Development of thrombosis while on heparin therapy is not always due to an insufficient dose or form of heparin.
3. Low-molecular-weight heparins and warfarin should not be used to treat patients with HIT.
4. Lepirudan (Refludan) or argatroban should be used to treat patients with HIT.
5. The clinician should consider routinely monitoring the platelet count every third day in all patients receiving heparin and should discontinue heparin if the platelet count drops to half of baseline.

REFERENCES

1. Warkentin TE, Levine MN, Hirsh J, et al: Heparin-induced thrombocytopenia in patients treated with low molecular weight heparin or unfractioned heparin. N Engl J Med 332:1330–1335, 1995.
2. Warkentin TE, Elavathil LJ, Hayward CP, et al: The pathogenesis of venous limb gangrene associated with heparin-induced thrombocytopenia. Ann Intern Med 127:804–812, 1997.
3. Warkentin TE, Kelton JG: Temporal aspects of heparin-induced thrombocytopenia. N Engl J Med 344:1286–1292, 2001.

PATIENT 74

A 79-year-old woman with rheumatoid arthritis and postoperative respiratory failure

A 79-year-old woman with a 50-year history of polyarticular, degenerative rheumatoid arthritis is referred for evaluation of acute respiratory failure after radical cystectomy for transitional cell carcinoma of the bladder. Preoperatively, her voice was normal, and she had mild restrictive lung disease, ischemic cardiomyopathy with a left ventricular ejection fraction of 40%, and a fixed inferior perfusion defect but no reversible defects on dipyridamole-thallium cardiac stress testing, and 3 mm of subluxation of C3 on C4 with neck flexion (see Figure). She was nasotracheally intubated and tolerated surgery well. Within minutes of extubation, she became acutely stridulous and tachypneic and required emergent reintubation.

Physical Examination: Temperature 98.9°F, pulse 105 and regular, respirations 10 (ventilated), blood pressure 110/70. Skin: no lesions. HEENT: normal. Lungs: before reintubation: inspiratory and exhalatory "wheezing," with poor air movement; after reintubation: clear to auscultation. Heart: regular tachycardia without new murmurs or gallops. Abdomen: normal. Extremities: no edema. Neuromuscular: no focal motor deficit, following simple commands.

Laboratory Findings: CBC: normal. EKG: sinus tachycardia, otherwise unchanged from preoperative. ABG: intermittent mandatory ventilation 10/min, pressure support 10 cm H_2O, PEEP 5 cm H_2O, FIO_2 100% pH 7.23, PCO_2 45 mmHg, PO_2 329 mmHg, calculated bicarbonate 19 mEq/L. Chest radiograph: no acute changes. Neck radiograph: see Figure.

Questions: What is the most likely cause of this patient's respiratory failure? What therapy should be instituted?

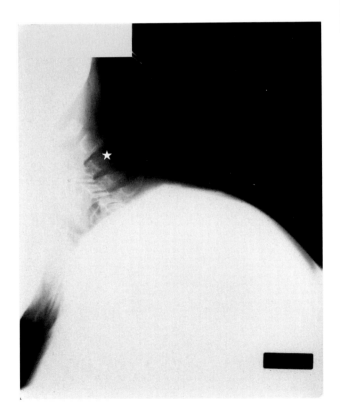

Answers: Acute laryngeal obstruction caused by vocal cord laxity from chronic rheumatoid degeneration of the cricoarytenoid cartilages, exacerbated by vocal cord swelling secondary to intubation. Initial therapy should be reintubation or, if necessary, emergent tracheotomy. Subsequent treatment might include a brief course of high-dose intravenous steroid to reduce laryngeal edema.

Discussion: Patients with rheumatoid arthritis are at risk for specific perioperative complications because of the manifestations of the disease and because of the medications used to treat it. Because rheumatoid arthritis can lead to destruction of the joints, it is crucial to assess the cervical spine before endotracheal intubation of a patient with rheumatoid arthritis. Forced extension of the neck during endotracheal intubation can cause subluxation of the cervical spine with consequent spinal cord injury. Although many patients would not benefit from radiography, patients with destructive joint disease, even if only of a few years' duration; patients with neck pain or posterior head pain; patients with limited neck mobility; and patients with distal neurologic symptoms possibly caused by spinal cord disease should be assessed further by plain radiography of the neck with flexion-extension views. Neurologic signs plus anterior atlantoaxial subluxation of >5 mm and mild vertical or posterior atlantoaxial subluxation generally are considered evidence of significant cervical spine instability that might require surgical stabilization or at least special approaches to intubation, such as nasotracheal or fiberoptic intubation, plus external cervical spine immobilization in the perioperative period. When in doubt, the clinician should refer the rheumatoid arthritis patient with significant neurologic symptoms and signs or abnormal plain radiography of the neck for evaluation by a neurologist or neurosurgeon.

As in the present patient, the cricoarytenoid joints can be damaged by rheumatoid inflammation, leading to relative vocal cord laxity. Especially with a traumatic or a prolonged endotracheal intubation, the larynx can swell and obstruct the airway. If a preoperative patient with rheumatoid arthritis is stridulous or chronically hoarse, the clinician should consider consulting an otolaryngologist before surgery to assess whether steroid injections or preoperative tracheotomy is indicated. In the patient with rheumatoid arthritis who is dyspneic after surgery, laryngeal obstruction should be considered.

The cardiopulmonary manifestations of rheumatoid arthritis should be evaluated preoperatively. These include, but are not limited to, pericardial effusion, pericardial fibrosis, myocardial fibrosis with consequent conduction system disease, and pleural effusion or pulmonary interstitial fibrosis with consequent restrictive lung disease. Clinically silent pericardial disease occurs in 45% of patients with rheumatoid arthritis. A patient's functional capacity frequently is limited by arthritis, making it difficult to assess cardiopulmonary reserve. In addition to a careful history and physical examination, ECG and chest radiography are indicated in most patients with rheumatoid arthritis. Additional cardiac (e.g., echocardiography, stress testing) and pulmonary testing (e.g., spirometry) might be indicated to assess cardiopulmonary reserve adequately in patients disabled by arthritis.

Many rheumatologists prefer to discontinue methotrexate 1 week before surgery and to restart it 1 week afterward. One small study showed a decreased risk of postoperative infection and no flares of arthritis in patients who discontinued taking methotrexate 1 week before surgery compared with patients who continued methotrexate throughout the perioperative period. A larger, prospective, randomized trial showed no apparent benefit of discontinuing methotrexate 2 weeks before surgery and restarting it 2 weeks after surgery.

To reduce perioperative blood loss and to reduce the risk of perioperative renal dysfunction, aspirin can be discontinued 1 week before surgery, and most other nonsteroidal antiinflammatory drugs, including cyclooxygenase-2 inhibitors (celecoxib [Celebrex], rofecoxib [Vioxx]) can be discontinued 2 to 3 days before to surgery. In the few days that the patient is not taking her or his usual nonsteroidal antiinflammatory drug, adequate analgesia usually can be achieved with acetaminophen alone or in combination with an opiate.

Steroid medications should be continued at the patient's usual dose until the day of surgery. For procedures involving only minor physiologic stress, the patient's usual dose of steroid should be continued throughout the perioperative period; however, for more stressful procedures, supplemental steroid is indicated. Patients taking ≤5 mg/d of prednisone usually do not require steroid supplementation. Patients taking >5 mg/d of prednisone might have suppression of the hypothalamic-pituitary-adrenal axis and should receive supplemental steroid for stressful procedures. If a patient taking ≥5 mg/d of prednisone develops perioperative complications, he or she also might benefit from supplemental steroid. For a procedure involving minor stress, such as inguinal herniorraphy, a single dose of hydrocortisone hemisuccinate, 25 mg intramuscularly, or methylprednisolone, 5 mg intravenously, at the start of surgery should be adequate. For a more stressful procedure, such as cholecystectomy or hemicolectomy, hydrocortisone hemisuccinate, 50 mg intravenously every 8 hours, or methylprednisolone, 10 mg intravenously every 6 hours, starting at the time of surgery and tapered over 1 to 2 days should be adequate. For major surgery such as major cardiothoracic or abdominal surgery, hydrocortisone hemisuccinate, 100 mg intravenously every 8 hours, or methylprednisolone, 20 mg intravenously every 6 hours, tapered over 2 to 3 days, should be adequate. The clinician should consider adrenal insufficiency in patients who are not currently taking steroid but have done so for more than 2 weeks at any time in the past year. Steroid therapy should be minimized to minimize consequent osteoporosis, glucose intolerance, and other associated adverse effects. If time permits, the clinician should consider testing the patient's hypothalamic-pituitary-adrenal axis with an adrenocorticotropic hormone stimulation test to determine if stress-dose steroid is needed.

In the present patient, the radiograph of the neck showed 3 mm of C3 on C4 (see Figure). The patient underwent tracheotomy and was extubated successfully the day after surgery. She was treated with hydrocortisone hemisuccinate, initially at 50 mg intravenously every 8 hours, tapered over 3 days to her usual prednisone, 10 mg orally once a day. Her voice returned to normal in 1 week.

Clinical Pearls

1. Plain radiography of the cervical spine should be obtained in preoperative patients with rheumatoid arthritis who have destructive joint disease, neck pain, limited neck mobility, or neurologic symptoms possibly caused by spinal cord disease.

2. Laryngeal swelling with obstruction should be included in the differential diagnosis of the patient with rheumatoid arthritis who is dyspneic after surgery.

3. Additional cardiac pulmonary testing should be considered to assess cardiopulmonary reserve adequately in patients disabled by arthritis.

4. Consider discontinuing methotrexate 1 week before surgery.

5. Consider stress-dose steroid for steroid-dependent patients undergoing major surgery or patients with severe perioperative complications.

REFERENCES

1. Carpenter MT, West SG, Vogelgesang SA, Casey Jones DE: Postoperative joint infections in rheumatoid arthritis patients on methotrexate therapy. Orthopedics 19:207–210, 1996.
2. Steuer A, Keat AC: Perioperative use of methotrexate—a survey of clinical practice. Br J Rheumatol 36:1009–1011, 1997.
3. Hamilton JD, Gordon MM, McInnes IB, et al: Improved medical and surgical management of cervical spine disease in patients with rheumatoid arthritis over 10 years. Ann Rheum Dis 59:434–438, 2000.
4. Grennan DM, Gray J, Loudon J, Fear S: Methotrexate and early postoperative complications in patients with rheumatoid arthritis undergoing elective orthopaedic surgery. Ann Rheum Dis 60:214–217, 2001.
5. Jabbour SA: Steroids and the surgical patient. Med Clin North Am 85:1311–1317, 2001.
6. Coursin DB, Wood KE: Corticosteroid supplementation for adrenal insufficiency. JAMA 287:236–240, 2002

PATIENT 75

A 29-year-old man with sickle cell anemia anticipating inguinal herniorraphy

A 29-year-old man with a history of sickle cell anemia presents for evaluation before elective inguinal herniorraphy. He has been hospitalized several times for painful sickling crises but has never had a stroke or a pulmonary infarction. He has not required blood transfusion in the past year and does not have RBC antibodies. His most recent painful crisis was 3 weeks before presentation. His only medication is folic acid, 1 mg orally daily.

Physical Examination: Temperature 98°F, pulse regular 66, respirations 12, blood pressure 117/55. Skin: no lesions. HEENT: normal. Lungs: clear to auscultation. Heart: regular rhythm with apical S_4 gallop and 2/6 crescendo murmur at left upper sternal border without radiation. Abdomen: liver edge percussed 3 cm below costal margin, spleen not palpable. Extremities: normal. Neuromuscular: normal.

Laboratory Findings: WBC 8,300/μL with normal differential, Hgb 9.4 g/dL, mean corpuscular volume 80 fL (normal range 88 to 97 fL), platelets 338,000/μL. BUN 9 mg/dL, creatinine 0.5 mg/dL. ECG: normal. Chest radiograph: borderline cardiomegaly, otherwise normal.

Question: What is this patient's risk for perioperative complications?

Answer: With proper care to minimize physiologic stressors that can precipitate sickling, he has a low risk (< 5%) for serious perioperative complications.

Discussion: Patients with sickle cell anemia, hemoglobin SC disease, and hemoglobin S/β-thalassemia are at high risk for perioperative complications, including infections, sickling crises, acute sickle chest syndrome, and death, because perioperative hypoxemia, hypothermia, dehydration, and acidosis can induce sickling, leading to vaso-occlusion and organ dysfunction. Most patients with sickle cell anemia are functionally asplenic, placing them at high risk for infections with encapsulated bacteria. The key to preventing a perioperative crisis is to minimize exposure to these situations. Appropriate measures include (1) administration of supplemental inhaled oxygen starting several hours before to surgery; (2) maintenance of normal body temperature (e.g., avoid exposing the extremities during surgery); (3) vigorous hydration starting several hours before surgery; (4) appropriate use of prophylactic antimicrobials; and (5) intraoperative ABG sampling as needed to monitor blood pH and oxygen content, especially during prolonged procedures.

Optimal transfusion therapy in the perioperative period for patients with sickle cell disease is unknown. The largest retrospective study showed an apparent benefit of perioperative RBC transfusion; however, the only prospective randomized trial showed that transfusing with the goal of reducing the sickle hemoglobin concentration to <30% was no better than transfusing only as needed to raise the total hemoglobin to 10 g/dL. The *Cochrane Database Review* concluded that although conservative transfusion practices seem to be generally as effective as more aggressive transfusion practices in the preparation of sickle cell patients for surgery, further research is needed.

Some patients with sickle cell anemia take hydroxyurea to reduce the frequency of sickling crises. Although there are no studies addressing this issue, it is reasonable to discontinue hydroxyurea a few days before surgery to minimize perioperative infection and to enable wound healing. Hydroxyurea can be restarted a few days after surgery, when initial wound healing is adequate.

A final preoperative consideration in patients with sickle cell anemia is that many have functional asplenia before reaching adulthood. This places them at risk for overwhelming sepsis from encapsulated organisms, such as pneumococcus and meningococcus. The preoperative evaluation is an opportunity to ensure appropriate vaccination coverage for these patients. Treatment of postoperative sickling crisis consists of (1) treating any hypoxemia, hypothermia, dehydration, infection, or acidosis; (2) transfusion of packed RBCs as needed; and (3) adequate pain control.

Before surgery, the present patient received pneumococcal vaccination, was transfused with 2 U of packed RBCs, and was vigorously hydrated intravenously. His oxygenation was maintained throughout the perioperative period. He experienced no sickling symptoms during hospitalization and tolerated herniorraphy without complications.

Clinical Pearls

1. Patients with sickle cell anemia are at increased risk for vaso-occlusive crisis if they are exposed to hypoxemia, hypothermia, dehydration, infection, or acidosis. These conditions must be avoided in the perioperative period; the clinician should consider using supplemental inhaled oxygen and vigorous intravenous hydration starting several hours before surgery.

2. The clinician should consider transfusing packed RBCs as needed to maintain hemoglobin >10 mg/dL.

3. The clinician should consider discontinuing hydroxyurea a few days before surgery and restarting it a few days after surgery when initial wound healing is adequate.

4. The preoperative evaluation is an opportunity to ensure appropriate vaccination coverage for patients with sickle cell anemia. The preoperative evaluation can be a crucial opportunity to administer important preventive care measures.

REFERENCES

1. Koshy M, Weiner SJ, Miller ST, et al: Surgery and anesthesia in sickle cell disease: Cooperative study of sickle cell diseases. Blood 86:3676–3684, 1995.
2. Vichinsky EP, Haberkern CM, Neumayr L, et al: A comparison of conservative and aggressive transfusion regimens in the perioperative management of sickle cell disease. N Engl J Med 333:206–213, 1995.
3. Riddlington C, Williamson L: Preoperative blood transfusions for sickle cell disease. Cochrane Database Syst Rev 3:CD003149, 2001.

INDEX

Abdominal distention, in postoperative ileus, 196–197
ACE inhibitors, see Angiotensin-converting enzyme inhibitors
ACTH, see Adrenocorticotropic hormone
Adrenal insufficiency
  causes, 205
  cholecystectomy patient, 204–206
  imaging, 205–206
  testing, 205
Adrenal suppression, evaluation in steroid-using patients, 67–69
Adrenocorticotropic hormone (ACTH)
  adrenal insufficiency testing, 205
  anesthesia and surgery response, 68
  stimulation testing, 69
Adynamic ileus, features, 196–197
Alcohol
  acute withdrawal syndrome, 139–141
  delirium tremens features, 141
  Revised Clinical Institute Withdrawal Assessment for Alcohol scale, 140
  seizure disorder in postoperative period, 180
Amiodarone, perioperative management, 156, 158
Anaphylaxis
  drug induction, 10
  intraoperative, 9–10
  postoperative cardiac arrest, 12
Anesthesia
  liver disease patients, 194
  malignant hyperthermia induction, 168
  risks in general versus regional anesthesia, 184–186
  seizure disorder patients, 179–180
  stroke risks, 165
  transurethral resection of the prostate, 183
Anesthetics, safety in pregnancy, 137–138
Angina, see Coronary artery disease
Angiotensin-converting enzyme (ACE) inhibitors
  hereditary angioneurotic edema as contraindication, 199
  pregnancy as contraindication, 122
  renal transplant recipients and surgery, 208
  surgical risks, 37
Anorexia nervosa
  cardiac manifestations, 102
  course, 101–103
  diagnostic criteria, 102
  endocrine abnormalities, 102
  epideiology, 102
  hospitalization criteria, 103
  medical clues, 102
  refeeding syndrome, 103
  treatment, 102–103

Antibiotics
  endocarditis prophylaxis, selection of antibiotic, 202–203
  prophylaxis with systolic click in urologic surgery, 93–94
  valvular heart disease prophylaxis, 43
Anticoagulation, management during surgery, 187–189
Anti-D antibody, idiopathic thrombocytopenic purpura management, 105
Aortic aneurysm
  hypertension in postoperative period, 71, 72
  preoperative risk evaluation, 54–56
Aortic stenosis, postoperative cardiac complications, 39–40, 43
Appendicitis, management in pregnancy, 136–138
Argatroban, heparin-induced thrombocytopenia management, 212
Arrhythmia, *see also specific arrhythmias*
  electrocardiography of perioperative arrhythmias, 19–20
  postoperative
    incidence, 81
    management, 81
    mechanisms, 81
    risk factors, 79, 81
Aspirin
  dental surgery patient management, 202, 203
  perioperative management, 156, 157, 215
Asthma
  perioperative complications, 26
  postoperative pulmonary complications, 24–27
  prevalence, 26
Atenolol, myocardial infarction, postoperative prevention, 143
Atorvastatin, perioperative management, 156
Atrial fibrillation
  perioperative anticoagulation management, 188
  postoperative arrhythmia risks and prevention, 79–81
  stroke risks, 166
Autonomic neuropathy
  assessment, 113, 114
  postoperative cardiac arrest, 12
  with postoperative respiratory arrest in diabetes, 112–114

Bacitracin, anaphylaxis, 10
Beta-agonists
  asthma management, 26, 116
  coronary artery disease with chronic obstructive pulmonary disease, surgical patient management, 90–91
  pregnancy safety, 116

Beta-blockers
  alcohol withdrawal syndrome management, 141
  arrhythmia management in postoperative period, 81
  coronary artery disease perioperative risk reduction, 33
  electroconvulsive therapy patient management, 49–50
  hypertensive patient perioperative management, 38
  mitral regurgitation patient perioperative management, 43–44
  myocardial infarction, postoperative prevention, 62, 143
  pain-induced hypertension management in postoperative period, 71–72
  perioperative management, 157
  pregnancy-induced hypertension management, 122–123
  rebound hypertension, 37
  surgical risk management 6 weeks after myocardial infarction, 59–60
  thyroid storm management, 6
  vascular surgery perioperative management, 55
Birth control, perioperative management, 157
Bisoprolol
  coronary artery disease perioperative risk reduction, 33
  postoperative prevention of myocardial infarction, 143
Bisphosphonates, perioperative management, 157

CABG, see Coronary artery bypass graft
CAD, see Coronary artery disease
Carbamazepine, diabetes insipidus management, 128
Carbidopa, infusion for NPO Parkinson's disease patients, 110
Carbon dioxide insufflation
  laparoscopic cholecystectomy, 30
  pregnant patients, 137
Cardiac arrest, postoperative, 11–12
Cardiac risk index
  Goldman index, 65
  guidelines for cardiac risk assessment, 65–66, 77, 91
  revised cardiac risk index, 65, 81
Cardiopulmonary bypass, postoperative neurologic dysfunction, 147–149
Carotid endarectomy, prophylactic, 165
Cataract
  preoperative risk assessment and management, 45–47
  surgery prevalence and complications, 46
Catecholamines, surgery response and hyperglycemia, 151
Celecoxib, perioperative management, 158
Cerebral aneurysm, hypertension following surgery, 98–100
Chest radiograph
  chronic obstructive pulmonary disease, 16, 21
  healthy surgical patient indications, 52–53
  respiratory infection, 73
Chlorpropamide, diabetes insipidus management, 128

Cholangitis, elderly patient preparation for surgery, 176–178
Cholecystectomy
  adrenal insufficiency patients, 204–206
  chest pain and electrocardiogram changes after surgery, 61–62
  laparoscopic versus open surgery complications, 28–32
  obese patient, 76–78
Choledocholithiasis, elderly patient preparation for surgery, 176–178
Chronic obstructive pulmonary disease (COPD)
  coronary artery disease comorbid surgical patient assessment, 90–91
  postoperative pulmonary complications, 16–17, 21–22
  surgical management of patients to reduce complications, 21–22
Cilostazol, perioperative management, 156, 157
Cirrhosis
  in alcoholics, 140
  Childs criteria for operative risk assessment
  postoperative hepatic encephalopathy, 193–195
  surgery risks, 194
CIWA scale, see Revised Clinical Institute Withdrawal Assessment for Alcohol scale
Clofibrate, diabetes insipidus management, 128
Clonidine, alcohol withdrawal syndrome management, 141
Clopidogrel, perioperative management, 157
Clostridium difficile
  diagnosis, 191
  diarrhea, 190–191
  risk factors for infection, 191
  toxins, 191
  treatment, 191
Computed tomography (CT)
  adrenal insufficiency evaluation, 205–206
  pulmonary embolism, 2
Confusion
  following cardiopulmonary bypass, 147–149
  donepezil for postoperative management, 177
  with hepatic encephalopathy, 193–194
  with hyponatremia, 85–87
  with neuroleptic malignant syndrome, 173–174
  after transurethral resection of the prostate, 181–183
Congestive heart failure
  diastolic dysfunction in postoperative period, 170–172
  postoperative cardiac complications, 43
COPD, see Chronic obstructive pulmonary disease
Coronary artery bypass graft (CABG), postoperative arrhythmia risks and prevention, 79–81
Coronary artery disease (CAD)
  chronic obstructive pulmonary disease comorbid surgical patient assessment, 90–91
  coronary revascularization in surgical risk reduction, 33
  perioperative complication reduction, 32–33
  peripheral vascular disease as indicator, 55

Coronary artery stenting, noncardiac surgery patient management, 107–108
Corticosteroids
  asthma management in preoperative period, 26–27
  perioperative steroid management, 67–69
  pregnancy safety
    inhaled steroids, 116–117
    systemic steroids, 117
  renal transplant recipients and surgery, 209–210
  rheumatoid arthritis perioperative management, 215–216
Cortisol
  adrenal insufficiency testing, 205
  normal levels, 205
Cricoarytenoid joints, rheumatoid arthritis degeneration, 215
Cromolyn sodium, pregnancy safety, 117
CT, see Computed tomography
Cyclosporine
  drug interactions, 209
  surgical considerations, 208

Dantrolene, malignant hyperthermia management, 168
Deep venous thrombosis (DVT)
  after gynecologic surgery, 2
  after major head and neck surgery, 210–213
  postoperative risk factors, 130–132
  in pregnancy, 118
  prophylaxis after previous occurrence, 88–89
  risk factors, 2
Delirium
  after hip repair, 160, 161
  definition, 134
  mental status testing, 134–135
  postoperative in elderly patients, 177, 178
  postoperative
    causes, 134
    risk factors, 134
    treatment, 135
Delirium tremens, features, 141
Dental surgery
  cyanotic heart disease patient, 201–203
  warfarin anticoagulation, 189
Depression electroconvulsive therapy risk assessment, 48–50
Diabetes
  autonomic neuropathy with postoperative respiratory arrest, 112–114
  cardiac and renal risks, 154
  gestational, see Gestational diabetes
  perioperative management of type 1 diabetes, 153–155
  postoperative hyperglycemia management in type 2 diabetes, 150–152
  postoperative ileus management, 196–197
  preoperative evaluation, 113, 114
Diabetes insipidus
  central causes, 128
  definition, 128
  postoperative, 127–129
  treatment, 128–129

Diarrhea
  Clostridium difficile, 190–191
  postoperative causes, 191
Digoxin
  perioperative management, 158
  toxicity risks and management, 171, 172
Dipyridamole, perioperative management, 157
Dipyridamole thallium testing
  safety, 91
  vascular surgery patient evaluation, 55–56, 91
Diuretics, surgical risks, 37
Dobutamine echocardiography, see Echocardiogram
Domperidone, Parkinson's disease postoperative management, 110
Donepezil, postoperative confusion management, 135, 177
Dopamine, intraoperative anaphylaxis management, 10
Dyspnea, see also Chronic obstructive pulmonary disease
  hypothyroidism and postoperative respiratory muscle weakening, 162–163
  with pulmonary embolism, 2
Dysrhythmia, postoperative cardiac arrest, 12

ECG, see Electrocardiogram
Echocardiogram
  anorexia nervosa, 102
  aortic stenosis, 39
  congestive heart failure, 171, 172
  dobutamine stress echocardiography, 55–56, 91
  mitral regurgitation, 43
  systolic click evaluation, 94
ECT, see Electroconvulsive therapy
Elderly patients
  demographic trends, 177
  nutrition, 177
  perioperative complications, 177–178
  physiology of aging, 177
  postoperative morbidity and mortality, 177
  preparation for surgery, 176–178
Electrocardiogram (ECG)
  anaphylaxis, 9–10
  anorexia nervosa, 102
  asthma in preoperative patient, 24–25
  atrial fibrillation, 80
  cataract surgery patient, 46
  cholecystectomy patient, preoperative evaluation, 28–29
  cyanotic heart disease patient before dental surgery, 202, 203
  healthy surgical patient indications, 52–53
  left ventricular hypertrophy, 35–36
  myocardial infarction
    postoperative, 61–62
    silent, 135
    surgical risk assessment 6 weeks after, 57–58
  perioperative arrhythmias, 19–20
  pulmonary embolism, 2
  transurethral resection of the prostate syndrome, 183
  vascular surgery patient evaluation, 55

Electrocautery, pacemaker management, 146
Electroconvulsive therapy (ECT)
    contraindications, 49
    risk assessment, 48–50
Endocarditis
    antibiotics for prophylaxis, 202–203
    prophylactic antibiotics with systolic click in uro-
        logic surgery, 93–94
    risk stratification, 202
Enflurane, seizure induction, 180
Ephedrine, intraoperative anaphylaxis management,
    10
Epidural anesthesia, risks, 185
Epinephrine, intraoperative anaphylaxis management,
    10

Fat embolism syndrome
    causes, 14
    following liver laceration repair, 13–15
    mortality, 14
Fever
    with fat embolism syndrome, 14
    with neuroleptic malignant syndrome, 173–174
    with respiratory infection, 73
    with thyroid storm, 4–5
Fondaparinux, deep venous thrombosis postoperative
    prophylaxis, 131
Furosemide, ascites management, 194

Garlic, bleeding risks with use, 8
Gastrectomy, cardiac risk assessment, 64–66
Gestational diabetes
    birth defects, 96, 97
    definition, 96
    hyperglycemia management, 96–97
    risk factors, 96
GFR, see Glomerular filtration rate
Ginkgo biloba, bleeding risks with use, 8
Ginseng, bleeding risks with use, 8
Glomerular filtration rate (GFR), renal transplant re-
    cipients and surgery, 208
Glucocorticoids, see Corticosteroids; Cortisol
α-Glucosidase inhibitors, perioperative management
    of diabetes, 151
Glycine toxicity, transurethral resection of the prostate
    syndrome, 182–183

HAE, see Hereditary angioneurotic edema
Haloperidol, postoperative delirium management, 135
HELLP syndrome, in pregnancy, 124–126
Hematocrit, healthy surgical patient indications, 53
Heparin
    antibody development incidence, 213
    deep venous thrombosis postoperative prophylaxis,
        131–132
    perioperative anticoagulation, 188, 189
    with regional anesthesia, 186
    thrombocytopenia induction, 89, 211–213
    thromboembolism management in pregnancy, 119,
        120

Hepatic encephalopathy, postoperative, 193–195
Hepatocellular carcinoma, perioperative mortality,
    195
Herbal supplements
    drug interactions, 8
    perioperative platelet dysfunction and bleeding,
        7–8
    preoperative discontinuation, 158
    prevalence of use, 8
Hereditary angioneurotic edema (HAE)
    fresh frozen plasma in preoperative period, 199
    pathophysiology, 199
    perioperative complication risks, 198–199
Hip fracture
    complications, 159–161
    delirium after repair, 160, 161
    epidemiology, 160
    osteoporosis evaluation, 161
    protein supplements in management, 160
    repair timing, 160
    types
        intertrochanteric fractures, 160
        intracapsular fractures, 160
        subtrochanteric fractures, 160
Hip replacement, deep venous thrombosis postopera-
    tive risk, 131
Hormone replacement therapy, perioperative
    management, 157
Hydralazine, hypertension management following
    cerebral aneurysm repair, 99
Hydrochlorothiazide, perioperative management, 156,
    157
Hydrocortisone
    perioperative steroid management, 69, 215–216
    thyroid storm management, 6
Hydroxyurea, perioperative management, 218
Hyperglycemia, see Diabetes
Hypertension
    blood pressure management in perioperative period,
        37–38
    cerebral aneurysm, hypertension following surgery,
        98–100
    diastolic dysfunction in postoperative period, 171
    pain induction in postoperative period, 70–72
    pheochromocytoma management in surgical
        patients, 83–84
    prevalence, 37
    surgical risk assessment, 35–38
Hyperthyroidism, see Thyroid storm
Hyponatremia
    postoperative features, 85–87
    serum osmolality and hyponatremia classification,
        86
    treatment
        hyovolemic hyponatremia, 86–87
        hypervolemic hyponatremia, 87
        hypotonic hyponatremia, 86
    in transurethral resection of the prostate syndrome,
        182, 183
Hypotension, from intraoperative anaphylaxis, 9–10

Hypothyroidism, postoperative respiratory muscle weakening, 162–163
Hypoxemia
  Parkinson's disease patients, 110
  postoperative, 163
Hysterectomy
  renal transplant patient, 207–209
  respiratory distress after, 1–2

ICD, see Implantable cardioverter-defibrillator
Idiopathic thrombocytopenic purpura (ITP), splenectomy management, 104–106
Ileus, postoperative, 196–197
Immunosuppresants, surgical considerations, 208–209
Implantable cardioverter-defibrillator (ICD), intraoperative management, 146
Infection, see Clostridium difficile; Endocarditis; Wound infection
Inferior vena cava filter, deep venous thrombosis prophylaxis, 89
Insulin
  gestational diabetes management, 96, 97
  perioperative management of type 1 diabetes, 153–155
Ipratropium, pregnancy safety, 116
ITP, see Idiopathic thrombocytopenic purpura

Ketamine, seizure induction, 180
Knee replacement, deep venous thrombosis postoperative risk and prophylaxis, 130–132

Labetalol
  hypertension management following cerebral aneurysm repair, 99
  pregnancy-induced hypertension management, 122–123
Lepirudan, heparin-induced thrombocytopenia management, 212
Leukotriene antagonists, pregnancy safety, 117
Levodopa, infusion for NPO Parkinson's disease patients, 110
Levothyroxine
  hypothyroidism management, 163
  perioperative management, 156, 158
Lisinopril, perioperative management, 156, 157
Liver function, third trimester of pregnancy, 125–126
Liver laceration repair, with fat embolism syndrome, 13–15
Lorazepam, alcohol withdrawal syndrome management, 140
Lugol solution, thyroid storm management, 6

Magnetic resonance imaging (MRI)
  adrenal insufficiency evaluation, 205–206
  electroconvulsive therapy risk assessment, 48
Malignant hyperthermia
  anesthetic induction, 168
  drug safety, 168
  incidence, 168
  intraoperative hemodynamic instability, 167–168
  treatment, 168

Meperidine, selegilene interactions, 111
Metformin, perioperative management of diabetes, 151
Methotrexate, perioperative management, 215, 216
Methyldopa, pregnancy-induced hypertension management, 123
Metronidazole, Clostridium difficile infection management, 191
Mitral regurgitation
  perioperative risks, 42–44
  prophylactic antibiotics with systolic click in urologic surgery, 93–94
  prosthetic valve patient anticoagulation management during surgery, 187–189
Mitral stenosis, perioperative risks, 43–44
Mivazerol, myocardial infarction, postoperative prevention, 143
MRI, see Magnetic resonance imaging
Myocardial infarction
  following coronary artery stenting, 108
  postoperative
    cardiac arrest, 12
    cholecystectomy, 61–62
    mortality, 62
    prevention, 142–143
  surgical risks 6 weeks after myocardial infarction, 57–60

Nedocromil, pregnancy safety, 117
Neuroleptic malignant syndrome (NMS)
  clinical presentation, 173–175
  differential diagnosis, 174
  mortality, 174
  pathophysiology, 174, 175
  treatment, 174
Nimodipine, hypertension management following cerebral aneurysm repair, 99
NMS, see Neuroleptic malignant syndrome

Obesity
  cholecystectomy risks, 76–78
  obstructive sleep apnea, 77
  perioperative outcome influences, 76–78
Obstructive sleep apnea, obese patient perioperative management, 77
Ondesetron, Parkinson's disease postoperative management, 110
Oxazepam, alcohol withdrawal syndrome management, 140

Pacemaker
  intraoperative management, 145–146
  magnet effects, 146
  resetting by electrocautery, 146
Pain, hypertension induction in postoperative period, 70–72
Parkinson's disease, postoperative worsening, 109–111
PE, see Pulmonary embolism
Percutaneous transluminal coronary angioplasty

(PTCA), noncardiac surgery patient management, 107–108
Petechia, with fat embolism syndrome, 13–15
Phenoxybenzamine, pheochromocytoma patient management, 84
Pheochromocytoma
    hypertension management in surgical patients, 83–84
    surgical resection, 84
    triad of symptoms, 84
Pindolol, pregnancy-induced hypertension management, 122–123
Pituitary adenoma
    management, 129
    postoperative diabetes insipidus, 127–129
Platelet transfusion, idiopathic thrombocytopenic purpura splenectomy patients, 104–105
Polymyalgia rheumatica, perioperative steroid management, 67–69
Preeclampsia
    clinical presentation, 122
    with elevated liver enzymes, 125, 126
Pregnancy
    acute fatty liver of pregnancy, 125
    appendicitis management, 136–138
    asthma management and drug safety, 115–117
    cholestasis of pregnancy, 125, 126
    deep venous thrombosis, 119
    diabetes, see Gestational diabetes
    HELLP syndrome, 124–126
    hypertension management, 121–123
    intraoperative management, 137–138
    laparoscopic surgery, 137
    pulmonary embolism, 118–120
    testing, healthy surgical patient indications, 53
Preventricular contractions (PVCs)
    with anorexia nervosa, 103
    perioperative arrhythmias, 19–20
Propanolol, thyroid storm management, 6
Propylthiouracil, thyroid storm management, 6
Prostate
    benign hypertrophy incidence, 182
    resction, see Transurethral resection of the prostate
Prosthetic heart valve, anticoagulation management during surgery, 187–189
PTCA, see Percutaneous transluminal coronary angioplasty
Pulmonary embolism (PE)
    after gynecologic surgery, 2
    postoperative cardiac arrest, 12
    in pregnancy, 118–120
    risk factors, 2
PVCs, see Preventricular contractions

Raloxifene, perioperative management, 156, 157, 158
Refeeding syndrome, management, 103
Renal transplant recipients
    hysterectomy patient, 207–209
    perioperative risks, 208–209

Repaglinide, perioperative management of diabetes, 151
Respiratory arrest, autonomic neuropathy with postoperative respiratory arrest in diabetes, 112–114
Respiratory infection, elective surgery guidelines, 73–74
Revised Clinical Institute Withdrawal Assessment for Alcohol (CIWA) scale, 140
Rheumatoid arthritis
    cardiopulmonary manifestations, 215
    drug management, 215–216
    perioperative complications, 215
    respiratory failure after bladder surgery, 214–216
Right bundle-branch block, perioperative arrhythmias, 19–20
Risperidone, postoperative delirium management, 135
Rofecoxib, perioperative management, 158

Seizure, perioperative risks, 179–180
Selegilene, meperidine interactions, 111
SIADH, see Syndrome of inappropriate antidiuretic hormone
Sickle cell disease
    infection risks, 218
    perioperative complications and prevention, 217–218
    transfusion therapy, 218
Smoking, cessation before surgery, 22
Spinal headache, features, 185, 186
Spirometry, chronic obstructive pulmonary disease, preoperative evaluation, 17, 22
Splenectomy
    for idiopathic thrombocytopenic purpura, 104–106
    infection rate in postoperative period, 106
    laparoscopy, 105
Stanozolol, iron malabsorption induction, 199
Stroke
    with cardiopulmonary bypass, 148, 149
    after general surgery, 165
    perioperative risk factors, 164–166
    postoperative timing, 165
Subarachnoid hemorrhage, cerebral aneurysm repair and hypertension, 98–100
Sulfonylureas, perioperative management of diabetes, 151
Syndrome of inappropriate antidiuretic hormone (SIADH)
    cerebral aneurysm repair and hypertension, 99
    hypothyroid patients, 163
    postoperative hyponatremia, 86, 87

Tachycardia
    with congestive heart failure, 170
    with hyponatremia, 85–87
    with malignant hyperthermia, 167–168
    with pulmonary embolism, 1–2
    with thyroid storm, 4–6
Theophylline, pregnancy safety, 117
Thiamine deficiency, Wernicke's encephalopathy, 140

Thiazolidinediones, perioperative management of diabetes, 151
Thrombocytopenia
  causes, 211
  heparin induction, 89, 211–213
  splenectomy for idiopathic thrombocytopenic purpura, 104–106
Thyroid storm
  after cesarean section, 4–6
  point system for diagnosis, 5
  treatment, 6
Ticlopidine, perioperative management, 157
Total parenteral nutrition, insulin in diabetes management, 155
Toxic megacolon, incidence and mortality, 191
Transphenoidal surgery, postoperative diabetes insipidus, 127–129
Transurethral resection of the prostate (TURP)
  anesthesia, 183
  complications, 182
  confusion after surgery, 181–183
  irrigating solutions, 182
  prophylactic antibiotics with systolic click, 93–94
  syndrome features, 182–183

Trihexyphenidyl, Parkinson's disease postoperative management, 110
Triple H therapy, hypertension management following cerebral aneurysm repair, 99
TURP, see Transurethral resection of the prostate

Vasopressin, diabetes insipidus management, 128–129
Vitamin E, bleeding risks with use, 8
Vitamin K, antiocoagulation reversal, 189, 194

Warfarin
  deep venous thrombosis postoperative prophylaxis, 131
  dental surgery patients, 189
  pregnancy as contraindication, 120
  preoperative discontinuation, 188, 189
  rebound phenomenon, 188
  vitamin E interactions, 8
Wernicke's encephalopathy, thiamine deficiency, 140
Wound infection, obese patient surgical risks, 77, 78

Ximelagatran, deep venous thrombosis postoperative prophylaxis, 131